Underground Clinical Vignettes
Vignettes
Psychiatry

FOURTH EDITION

Underground Clinical Vignettes

Psychiatry

FOURTH EDITION

Sandra I. Kim, M.D., Ph.D.
Resident in Internal Medicine
Beth Israel Deaconess Medical Center
Harvard Medical School
Boston, Massachusetts

Todd A. Swanson, M.D., Ph.D.
Resident in Radiation Oncology
William Beaumont Hospital
Royal Oak, Michigan

Jason P. Caplan, M.D.
Clinical Fellow in Psychiatry
Massachusetts General Hospital
Harvard Medical School
Boston, Massachusetts

Wolters Kluwer | Lippincott Williams & Wilkins
Health
Philadelphia · Baltimore · New York · London
Buenos Aires · Hong Kong · Sydney · Tokyo

Acquisitions editor: Nancy Anastasi Duffy
Developmental editor: Nancy Hoffmann
Managing editor: Kelly Horvath
Production editor: Kevin Johnson
Marketing manager: Jennifer Kuklinski
Designer: Doug Smock
Compositor: International Typesetting and Composition

WM
18.2
P974
2007

© 2007 by Lippincott Williams & Wilkins
UCV Step 2 Psychiatry, . . .

Lippincott Williams & Wilkins, a Wolters Kluwer business.

351 West Camden Street   530 Walnut Street
Baltimore, MD 21201   Philadelphia, PA 19106

9 8 7 6 5 4 3 2 1

Library of Congress Cataloging-in-Publication Data

Kim, Sandra.
    Psychiatry / Sandra I. Kim, Todd A. Swanson, Jason P. Caplan.—4th ed.
        p. ; cm.—(Underground clinical vignettes)
    Includes index.
    Rev. ed. of: Psychiatry / Vikas Bhushan . . . [et al.]. 3rd ed. 2005.
    ISBN-13: 978-0-7817-6846-7
    ISBN-10: 0-7817-6846-2
    1. Psychiatry—Case studies.   2. Physicians—Licenses—United
States—Examinations—Study guides.   I. Swanson, Todd A.   II. Caplan,
Jason P.   III. Psychiatry.   IV. Title.   V. Series.
    [DNLM: 1. Mental Disorders—Case Reports.   2. Mental
Disorders—Problems and Exercises.   WM 18.2 K49p 2007]
    RC465.B526 2007
    616.890076—dc22

                                                    2007033843

DISCLAIMER

dedication

Dedicated to the patients we care for.

preface

First published in 1999, the *Underground Clinical Vignettes* (UCV) series has provided thousands of students with a highly effective review tool as they prepare for medical examinations, particularly the USMLE Step 1 and 2 examinations. Designed as a quick study guide, each UCV book contains patient-centered clinical cases that highlight a range of medical diagnoses.

With this new edition of Step 2 UCV, we have incorporated feedback from medical students across the country to provide updated cases with expanded treatment and discussion sections. Every title has more cases, drawing from a broader area within each discipline. A new two-page format enables readers to formulate an initial diagnosis prior to reading the "answer" to each case. The inclusion of relevant magnetic resonance images, x-rays, and photographs allows students to more readily visualize the physical presentation of each case. Breakout point, tables, and algorithms have been added, along with 20 all-new, board-format questions-and-answers, making this edition of UCV an ideal source of information for examination review, classroom discussion, and clinical rotations.

The clinical vignettes in this Step 2 series have been revised and updated to reflect current medical thinking on medication, pathogenesis, epidemiology, management, and complications. Although each case presents most of the signs, symptoms, and diagnostic findings for a particular illness, patients typically do not present with such a "complete" picture, either clinically or on a medical examination. Cases are not meant to simulate a potential real patient or an examination vignette.

Access to Lippincott Williams & Wilkins (LWW)'s online companion site, ThePoint, is offered as a premium with the purchase of the UCV Step 2 bundle. Benefits include an online test link and 160 additional new board-format questions covering all UCV subject areas.

We hope you will find the UCV series informative and useful. We welcome any feedback, suggestions, or corrections you have about this series. Please contact us at LWW.com/medstudent.

contributors

Series Editors

Sandra I. Kim, M.D., Ph.D.
Resident in Internal Medicine
Beth Israel Deaconess Medical Center
Harvard Medical School
Boston, Massachusetts

Todd A. Swanson, M.D., Ph.D.
Resident in Radiation Oncology
William Beaumont Hospital
Royal Oak, Michigan

Book Editor

Jason P. Caplan, M.D.
Assistant Professor of Clinical Psychiatry
Director of Consultation Psychiatry
University Physicians Health Care
Kino Hospital
Tucsen, Arizona

Contributing Editor

Carrie E. Milligan, M.D.
Clinical Instructor in Psychiatry
Beth Israel Deaconess Medical Center
Harvard Medical School
Boston, Massachusetts

Contributors

Jane E. Caplan, M.D.
Rebecca Pace Barclay, M.D.
Jason B. Strauss, M.D.
Craigan P. Usher, M.D.

acknowledgments

Our great thanks to the house staff and faculty from Beth Israel Deaconess, Massachusetts General, Brigham and Women's, and Children's Hospitals in Boston, whose clinical cases, revisions, and suggestions were indispensable to this series. Thanks to the editors at Lippincott Williams & Wilkins, especially Nancy Hoffmann, who worked overtime on these books.

abbreviations

A-a	alveolar-arterial (oxygen gradient)	ATLS	Advanced Trauma Life Support (protocol)
AAA	abdominal aortic aneurysm	ATN	acute tubular necrosis
ABCs	airway, breathing, circulation	ATPase	adenosine triphosphatase
ABGs	arterial blood gases	ATRA	all-*trans*-retinoic acid
ABPA	allergic bronchopulmonary aspergillosis	AV	arteriovenous, atrioventricular
ABVD	Adriamycin, bleomycin, vinblastine, dacarbazine (chemotherapy)	AVPD	avoidant personality disorder
		AXR	abdominal x-ray
ACE	angiotensin-converting enzyme	AZT	azidothymidine (zidovudine)
ACTH	adrenocorticotropic hormone	BCG	bacille Calmette-Guérin
ADA	adenosine deaminase, American Diabetic Association	BE	barium enema
		BP	blood pressure
ADH	antidiuretic hormone	BPD	borderline personality disorder
ADHD	attention-deficit hyperactivity disorder	BPH	benign prostatic hypertrophy
		BPK	B-cell progenitor kinase
AED	automatic external defibrillator	BPM	beats per minute
AFP	α-fetoprotein	BUN	blood urea nitrogen
AI	aortic insufficiency	CAA	cerebral amyloid angiopathy
AICD	automatic internal cardiac defibrillator	CABG	coronary artery bypass grafting
		CAD	coronary artery disease
AIDS	acquired immunodeficiency syndrome	CALLA	common acute lymphoblastic leukemia antigen
ALL	acute lymphocytic leukemia	C-ANCA	cytoplasmic antineutrophil cytoplasmic antibody
ALS	amyotrophic lateral sclerosis		
ALT	alanine aminotransferase	CAO	chronic airway obstruction
AMA	American Medical Association	CAP	community-acquired pneumonia
AML	acute myelogenous leukemia	CBC	complete blood count
AMP	adenosine monophosphate	CBD	common bile duct
ANA	antinuclear antibody	CBT	cognitive behavioral therapy
ANCA	antineutrophil cytoplasmic antibody	CCU	cardiac care unit
		CD	cluster of differentiation
Angio	angiography	CDC	Centers for Disease Control and Prevention
AP	anteroposterior		
aPTT	activated partial thromboplastin time	CEA	carcinoembryonic antigen
		CF	cystic fibrosis
ARDS	adult respiratory distress syndrome	CFTR	cystic fibrosis transmembrane regulator
ARF	acute renal failure	CFU	colony-forming unit
AS	ankylosing spondylitis	CHF	congestive heart failure
5-ASA	5-aminosalicylic acid	CJD	Creutzfeldt–Jakob disease
ASA	acetylsalicylic acid	CK	creatine kinase
ASD	atrial septal defect	CK-MB	creatine kinase, MB fraction
ASO	antistreptolysin O	CLL	chronic lymphocytic leukemia
AST	aspartate aminotransferase	CML	chronic myelogenous leukemia

CMV	cytomegalovirus	E:I	expiratory-to-inspiratory (ratio)
CN	cranial nerve	ELISA	enzyme-linked immunosorbent assay
CNS	central nervous system		
CO	cardiac output	EM	electron microscopy
COPD	chronic obstructive pulmonary disease	EMG	electromyography
		ER	emergency room
CPAP	continuous positive airway pressure	ERCP	endoscopic retrograde cholangiopancreatography
CPK	creatine phosphokinase	ESR	erythrocyte sedimentation rate
CPR	cardiopulmonary resuscitation	EtOH	ethanol
CRP	C-reactive protein	FDA	Food and Drug Administration
CSF	cerebrospinal fluid	Fe_{Na}	fractional excretion of sodium
CT	computed tomography	FEV_1	forced expiratory volume in 1 second
CVA	cerebrovascular accident		
CXR	chest x-ray	FIGO	International Federation of Gynecology and Obstetrics (classification)
D&C	dilatation and curettage		
DAF	decay-accelerating factor		
DC	direct current	Flo_2	fraction of inspired oxygen
DEXA	dual-energy x-ray absorptiometry	FNA	fine-needle aspiration
DHEA	dehydroepiandrosterone	FRC	functional residual capacity
DIC	disseminated intravascular coagulation	FSH	follicle-stimulating hormone
		FTA	fluorescent treponemal antibody
DIP	distal interphalangeal (joint)	FTA-ABS	fluorescent treponemal antibody absorption test
DKA	diabetic ketoacidosis		
DL_{co}	diffusing capacity of carbon monoxide	5-FU	5-fluorouracil
		FVC	forced vital capacity
DM	diabetes mellitus	G6PD	glucose-6-phosphate dehydrogenase
DMD	Duchenne's muscular dystrophy		
DNA	deoxyribonucleic acid	GA	gestational age
DNase	deoxyribonuclease	GABA	gamma-aminobutyric acid
dsDNA	double-stranded DNA	GABHS	group A β-hemolytic streptococcus
DSM-IV	Diagnostic and Statistical Manual of Mental Disorders, Fourth edition		
		GAD	generalized anxiety disorder
		GBM	glomerular basement membrane
DTP	diphtheria, tetanus, pertussis (vaccine)	G-CSF	granulocyte colony-stimulating factor
DTRs	deep tendon reflexes	GERD	gastroesophageal reflux disease
DTs	delirium tremens	GFR	glomerular filtration rate
DUB	dysfunctional uterine bleeding	GGT	gamma-glutamyltransferase
DVT	deep venous thrombosis	GI	gastrointestinal
EBV	Epstein–Barr virus	GnRH	gonadotropin-releasing hormone
ECG	electrocardiography	GU	genitourinary
Echo	echocardiography	HAV	hepatitis A virus
ECMO	extracorporeal membrane oxygenation	Hb	hemoglobin
		HBcAg	hepatitis B core antigen
ECT	electroconvulsive therapy	HBsAg	hepatitis B surface antigen
EDTA	ethylenediamine tetraacetic acid	HBV	hepatitis B virus
EEG	electroencephalography	hCG	human chorionic gonadotropin
EF	ejection fraction	HCl	hydrogen chloride
EGD	esophagogastroduodenoscopy	HCO_3	bicarbonate

Hct	hematocrit	JVP	jugular venous pressure
HCV	hepatitis C virus	KOH	potassium hydroxide
HDL	high-density lipoprotein	KS	Kaposi's sarcoma
HEENT	head, eyes, ears, nose, and throat	KUB	kidney, ureters, bladder
HELLP	hemolysis, elevated liver enzymes, low platelets (syndrome)	LA	left atrium
		LAMB	lentigines, atrial myxoma, blue nevi (syndrome)
HEV	hepatitis E virus	LD	Leishman-Donovan (body)
HGPRT	hypoxanthine-guanine phospho-ribosyltransferase	LDH	lactate dehydrogenase
HHV	human herpesvirus	LDL	low-density lipoprotein
5-HIAA	5-hydroxyindoleacetic acid	LES	lower esophageal sphincter
HIDA	hepato-iminodiacetic acid (scan)	LFTs	liver function tests
HIV	human immunodeficiency virus	LH	luteinizing hormone
HLA	human leukocyte antigen	LHRH	luteinizing hormone–releasing hormone
HPF	high-power field		
HPI	history of present illness	LKM	liver-kidney microsomal (antibody)
HPV	human papillomavirus	LMN	lower motor neuron
HR	heart rate	LP	lumbar puncture
HRCT	high-resolution computed tomography	L/S	lecithin-to-sphingomyelin (ratio)
		LSD	lysergic acid diethylamide
HS	hereditary spherocytosis	LV	left ventricle, left ventricular
HSG	hysterosalpingography	LVH	left ventricular hypertrophy
HSV	herpes simplex virus	Lytes	electrolytes
HUS	hemolytic-uremic syndrome	Mammo	mammography
IABC	intra-aortic balloon counterpul-sation	MAO	monoamine oxidase (inhibitor)
		MAP	mean arterial pressure
ICA	internal carotid artery	MCA	middle cerebral artery
ICD	implantable cardiac defibrillator	MCHC	mean corpuscular hemoglobin concentration
ICP	intracranial pressure		
ICU	intensive care unit	MCP	metacarpophalangeal (joint)
ID/CC	identification and chief complaint	MCV	mean corpuscular volume
IDDM	insulin-dependent diabetes mellitus	MDMA	3,4-methylene-dioxymetham-phetamine ("Ecstasy")
IE	infectious endocarditis	MEN	multiple endocrine neoplasia
IFA	immunofluorescent antibody	MGUS	monoclonal gammopathy of undetermined origin
Ig	immunoglobulin		
IL	interleukin	MHC	major histocompatibility complex
IM	infectious mononucleosis, intramuscular	MI	myocardial infarction
		MIBG	metaiodobenzylguanidine
INH	isoniazid	MMR	measles, mumps, rubella (vaccine)
INR	International Normalized Ratio		
123-ISS	iodine-123-labeled somatostatin	MPTP	1-methyl-4-phenyl-tetrahydropy-ridine
IUD	intrauterine device		
IUGR	intrauterine growth retardation	MR	magnetic resonance (imaging)
IV	intravenous	mRNA	messenger ribonucleic acid
IVC	inferior vena cava	MRSA	methicillin-resistant *Staphylococcus aureus*
IVIG	intravenous immunoglobulin		
IVP	intravenous pyelography	MS	multiple sclerosis
JRA	juvenile rheumatoid arthritis	MTP	metatarsophalangeal (joint)
JVD	jugular venous distention	MuSK	muscle-specific kinase

MVA	motor vehicle accident
NADPH	reduced nicotinamide adenine dinucleotide phosphate
NAME	nevi, atrial myxoma, myxoid neurofibroma, ephilides (syndrome)
NG	nasogastric
NIDDM	noninsulin-dependent diabetes mellitus
NMDA	*N*-methyl-D-aspartate
NPO	nil per os (nothing by mouth)
NSAID	nonsteroidal anti-inflammatory drug
Nuc	nuclear medicine
OCD	obsessive-compulsive disorder
OCP	oral contraceptive pill
OCPD	obsessive-compulsive personality disorder
17-OHP	17-hydroxyprogesterone
OPC	organophosphate and carbamate
OS	opening snap
OTC	over the counter
PA	posteroanterior
2-PAM	pralidoxime
P-ANCA	perinuclear antineutrophil cytoplasmic antibody
Pao_2	partial pressure of oxygen
PAS	periodic acid Schiff
PBS	peripheral blood smear
Pco_2	partial pressure of carbon dioxide
PCOD	polycystic ovary disease
PCP	phencyclidine
PCR	polymerase chain reaction
PCV	polycythemia vera
PDA	patent ductus arteriosus
PE	physical exam
PEEP	positive end-expiratory pressure
PET	positron emission tomography
PFTs	pulmonary function tests
PID	pelvic inflammatory disease
PIP	proximal interphalangeal (joint)
PKU	phenylketonuria
PMI	point of maximal impulse
PMN	polymorphonuclear (leukocyte)
PO	per os (by mouth)
Po_2	partial pressure of oxygen
PPD	purified protein derivative
PROM	premature rupture of membranes
PRPP	phosphoribosyl pyrophosphate
PSA	prostate-specific antigen
PT	prothrombin time

PTE	pulmonary thromboembolism
PTH	parathyroid hormone
PTSD	post-traumatic stress disorder
PTT	partial thromboplastin time
RA	rheumatoid arthritis, right atrial
RBC	red blood cell
RDW	red-cell distribution width
REM	rapid eye movement
RF	rheumatoid factor
RhoGAM	Rh immune globulin
RNA	ribonucleic acid
RPR	rapid plasma reagin
RR	respiratory rate
RS	Reed-Sternberg (cell)
RSV	respiratory syncytial virus
RTA	renal tubular acidosis
RUQ	right upper quadrant
RV	residual volume, right ventricle, right ventricular
RVH	right ventricular hypertrophy
SA	sinoatrial
SAH	subarachnoid hemorrhage
Sao_2	oxygen saturation in arterial blood
SBE	subacute bacterial endocarditis
SBFT	small bowel follow-through
SC	subcutaneous
SCC	squamous cell carcinoma
SIADH	syndrome of inappropriate secretion of antidiuretic hormone
SIDS	sudden infant death syndrome
SLE	systemic lupus erythematosus
SMA	smooth muscle antibody
SSPE	subacute sclerosing panencephalitis
SSRI	selective serotonin reuptake inhibitor
STD	sexually transmitted disease
SZPD	schizoid personality disorder
T_3	triiodothyronine
T_4	thyroxine
TAB	therapeutic abortion
TB	tuberculosis
TBSA	total body surface area
TCA	tricyclic antidepressant
TCD	transcranial Doppler
TD	tardive dyskinesia
TENS	transcutaneous electrical nerve stimulation
TFTs	thyroid function tests
THC	*trans*-tetrahydrocannabinol

TIA	transient ischemic attack	UMN	upper motor neuron
TIBC	total iron-binding capacity	URI	upper respiratory infection
TIPS	transjugular intrahepatic portosystemic shunt	US	ultrasound
		UTI	urinary tract infection
TLC	total lung capacity	UV	ultraviolet
TMJ	temporomandibular joint (syndrome)	VCUG	voiding cystourethrogram
		VDRL	Venereal Disease Research Laboratory
TMP-SMX	trimethoprim-sulfamethoxazole		
TNF	tumor necrosis factor	VF	ventricular fibrillation
TNM	tumor, node, metastasis (staging)	VIN	vulvar intraepithelial neoplasia
ToRCH	*Toxoplasma,* rubella, CMV, herpes zoster	VLDL	very low density lipoprotein
		VMA	vanillylmandelic acid
tPA	tissue plasminogen activator	V/Q	ventilation-perfusion (ratio)
TPO	thyroid peroxidase	VS	vital signs
TRAP	tartrate-resistant acid phosphatase	VSD	ventricular septal defect
TRH	thyrotropin-releasing hormone	VT	ventricular tachycardia
TSH	thyroid-stimulating hormone	vWF	von Willebrand factor
TSS	toxic shock syndrome	VZIG	varicella-zoster immune globulin
TSST	toxic shock syndrome toxin		
TTP	thrombotic thrombocytopenic purpura	VZV	varicella-zoster virus
		WAGR	Wilms' tumor, aniridia, ambiguous genitalia, mental retardation (syndrome)
TUBD	transurethral balloon dilatation		
TUIP	transurethral incision of the prostate		
		WBC	white blood cell
TURP	transurethral resection of the prostate	WG	Wegener's granulomatosis
		WPW	Wolff–Parkinson–White (syndrome)
UA	urinalysis		
UGI	upper GI (series)	XR	x-ray

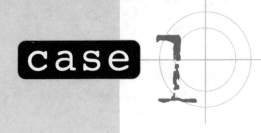

case 1

CC A **73-year-old woman** who had been doing well following an uncomplicated coronary artery bypass graft is now agitated and attempting to leave the hospital.

HPI She pulled off her telemetry leads this evening stating, "I'm not paying for another night in this hotel." When redirected back to her room, she became increasingly **agitated** and assaulted a nurse. Nursing staff note that the patient has become **increasingly confused over the past several hours.** She is **arousable and responsive** but has **difficulty attending** to simple tasks (eg, spelling WORLD backward). She is **unable to identify the date or city.** The chart reveals that the patient has had intermittent **periods of appearing quiet and withdrawn** since her surgery.

PE VS: fever (39.6°C); tachycardia (HR 105); normal BP; normal RR. PE: appropriate incisional tenderness.

Labs CBC: leukocytosis (13,000). Lytes: normal. BUN, creatinine, vitamin B_{12}, folate, and TFTs normal; RPR/VDRL nonreactive. UA: moderate bacteria and leukocyte-esterase positive; urine toxicology negative. Blood cultures pending.

Imaging CT, head: normal.

case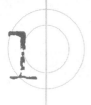

Delirium

Differential

Dementia is manifested in patients who are typically consistently alert. They do not show the lack of attention and acute waxing and waning course indicative of delirium.

Psychotic disorders involve consistent psychotic symptoms, whereas psychosis associated with delirium fluctuates with the level of consciousness.

Substance withdrawal delirium occurs in the setting of cessation of drug use (typically alcohol or sedative-hypnotics).

Pathogenesis

Delirium is a transient cognitive disorder characterized by disturbance of consciousness and change in cognition that **develop over a short period of time.** The course of delirium is marked by **waxing and waning of consciousness;** the patient appears alternately confused and alert. **Hallucinations and paranoia** may occur. By definition, **delirium is secondary to an underlying physiologic condition.** Anticholinergics, narcotics, benzodiazepines, and steroids are common agents that may result in **substance-induced delirium.** Common causes of **delirium due to a general medical condition** include infection, metabolic disturbance, and intracranial processes. **The elderly are particularly vulnerable to delirium** and can develop significant mental status changes from seemingly minor conditions. EEG in delirium shows **characteristic theta-delta slowing.**

Management

A **thorough medical evaluation** to identify and treat the underlying cause of delirium is critical. **Neuroleptics** (eg, haloperidol, olanzapine) are used to manage delirium, psychosis, and agitation. Withdrawal of potential deliriogenic medications is also advised. Benzodiazepines should be used only in the context of alcohol or sedative/hypnotic withdrawal, because they exacerbate delirium due to other causes. Serial mental status exams should be performed. Patients may require mechanical restraint and/or constant observation to reduce risk of self-harm.

Breakout Point

Life-Threatening Causes of Delirium (4H WIMPS)
Hypoxia/Hypoperfusion of the Brain
Hypertensive Crisis
Hypoglycemia
Hyper- or Hypothermia
Withdrawal/Wernicke Encephalopathy
Intracranial Bleed/Mass
Meningitis/Encephalitis
Poisons (including medications)
Status Epilepticus

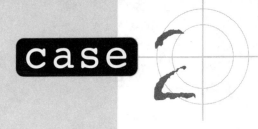

case

CC A **68-year-old** retired teacher is referred for psychiatric evaluation by her primary care physician for **progressive forgetfulness**.

HPI Her daughter notes that she has not been paying her bills on time and adds that she has seemed generally more **disorganized**. She frequently **loses things** and has gotten **lost** in her neighborhood on several occasions.

PE **Alert and oriented to person, place, and year;** unable to recall specific day and month; **long-term memory is intact** but **short-term memory is impaired;** patient has difficulty identifying objects **(agnosia)** and performing calculations; unable to perform three-stage commands or mimic complex hand gestures **(apraxia)**; at times, patient demonstrates difficulty generating normal speech **(aphasia)**; CN II through XII intact with normal motor and sensory function throughout.

Labs Lytes/CBC: normal. TFTs normal; RPR/VDRL nonreactive. UA: toxicology negative.

Imaging CT, head: **diffuse cerebral atrophy** without evidence of mass, infarct, or bleed.

case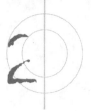

Dementia

Differential

Delirium is characterized by a gross impairment in consciousness, attention, and orientation with an acute onset and a course that fluctuates dramatically over hours or days.

Multi-infarct dementia results from repeated CNS infarctions of various sizes. The clinical course of vascular dementia is often characterized by a "stepwise" decline that is thought to correlate with each successive ischemic event.

Alcoholic dementia may be due to the neurotoxic effects of chronic use or an associated thiamine (vitamin B₁) deficiency.

Pick disease is characterized by frontal and temporal lobe atrophy.

Major depressive disorder can mimic dementia (**pseudodementia**).

Dementia due to general medical conditions may result from neoplasm, **normal pressure hydrocephalus**, demyelization illnesses, trauma, toxic encephalopathies, and infectious diseases (eg, HIV).

Pathogenesis

Dementia is caused by a variety of processes; Alzheimer dementia is the most common type and is associated with **neurofibrillary tangles, amyloid plaques,** and **degeneration of the nucleus basalis of Meynert.** Physiologically it is associated with **decreased central cholinergic transmission.** Risk factors include age, family history, and **homozygous apolipoprotein E ε4 alleles.**

Complications

Patients with significant dementia may develop delusions and hallucinations. Depression occurs in half of patients. In most dementias, deterioration occurs over 5 to 10 years, leading to death.

Management

Thorough medical evaluation is critical to **rule out underlying treatable causes of dementia.** Treatment for Alzheimer dementia is largely supportive, aimed at keeping the patient safe, educating the family, and increasing supervision as warranted. **Acetylcholinesterase inhibitors** (donepezil [Aricept] or rivastigmine [Exelon]) can temporarily augment central cholinergic transmission. Memantine, an NMDA antagonist, is approved for use in the advanced stages of disease. **Neuroleptics** are useful in the management of the agitated/psychotic dementia patient, although the atypical neuroleptics carry a black-box warning for sudden death in this population. Anticholinergic agents and benzodiazepines may cause further impairment of cognition.

Breakout Point

Conditions That May Mimic the Symptoms of Dementia (DEMENTIA)	
Drug Use	**T**umors/Trauma
Emotional Disorders	**I**nfection
Metabolic Disorders	**A**lcohol/Atherosclerosis
Eye and Ear Disorders	
Nutritional Disorders/Normal Pressure Hydrocephalus	

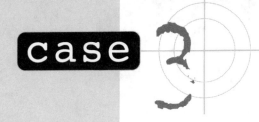

case

CC A 63-year-old man is brought to the ER by ambulance after having been found stumbling **drunk** downtown.

HPI The patient was admitted to the medical service for evaluation of **confusion that persisted despite resolution of his acute intoxication.** During hospitalization, he could not remember the names of his physicians (anterograde amnesia) or past events (retrograde amnesia) and often **fabricated answers to questions** (confabulation).

PE VS: normal. PE: hepatomegaly; **nystagmus**; polyneuropathy; impaired left lateral gaze (CN VI); **ataxia**.

Labs **CBC: macrocytic anemia.** Lytes/UA: normal. BUN and creatinine within normal limits. LFTs: AST and ALT elevated in a 2:1 ratio. **Serum thiamine pyrophosphate low.**

Imaging MR imaging, brain with hemorrhage in mammillary bodies.

case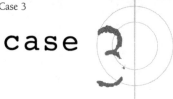

Wernicke-Korsakoff Syndrome

Differential

Acute intoxication from alcohol or other substances can be associated with the same nonspecific neurologic findings as Wernicke-Korsakoff syndrome; careful history and observation along with a toxicology screen is thus essential to diagnosis.

Alcohol withdrawal can lead to DTs (delirium, autonomic hyperactivity, and seizures); Wernicke-Korsakoff syndrome is not associated with autonomic instability and persists despite prolonged abstinence from alcohol.

Pathogenesis

Thiamine deficiency, in this case secondary to chronic alcoholism, is associated with CNS lesions located in the thalamus, hypothalamus, midbrain, pons, medulla, fornix, cerebellum, and mammillary bodies. **Wernicke encephalopathy** (characterized by **ataxia, ophthalmoplegia,** and **confusion**) may progress to **Korsakoff syndrome** (characterized by **amnesia** and **confabulation**). When both entities exist, a diagnosis of Wernicke-Korsakoff syndrome is made.

Management

Thiamine (vitamin B_1) IV administered daily for at least 3 days, with ongoing supplementation PO thereafter. Because glucose depletes thiamine stores, **thiamine administration should always precede glucose.** Treatment should be continued for 1 to 2 weeks for Wernicke encephalopathy and 3 to 12 months for Korsakoff syndrome. Prompt treatment of Wernicke encephalopathy may prevent progression to Korsakoff syndrome. Thiamine replacement may reverse ataxia, ophthalmoplegia, and nystagmus; however, amnesia and confusion do not respond as effectively to treatment, and full recovery of normal cognitive function is rare. Deficiencies of numerous other nutritional factors (including folate and vitamin B_{12} that lead to the characteristic macrocytic anemia) are also associated with alcohol abuse.

Breakout Point

Drinking Beer by the CAN May Lead to the Triad of Wernicke Encephalopathy
Confusion
Ataxia
Nystagmus (ophthalmoplegia)

case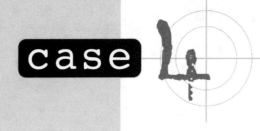

CC   An 86-year-old man is brought into the ER by his daughter who notes, "he keeps saying that he **sees spiders and snakes everywhere**. I think he's losing it."

HPI   Over the past few years, he has suffered **marked cognitive decline** and is now frequently **confused by his surroundings** and unable to perform simple tasks such as dressing and preparing meals for himself. He has experienced **difficulty walking** and he has fallen down three times in the past month without serious injury. He has no significant past medical history except for mild hypertension.

PE   VS: normal. Exam notable for **cogwheel rigidity** and **bradykinesia.** No resting tremor is appreciated.

Labs Not relevant.

Imaging MR imaging, head: normal.

Micropathology On expiration, the patient's autopsy pathology of the brain demonstrates intracytoplasmic inclusions with a dense core surrounded by a clear halo.

case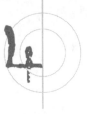

Lewy Body Dementia (LBD)

Differential

Alzheimer dementia is by far the most common form of dementia. Parkinsonism is usually not noted in patients with Alzheimer disease.

Parkinson disease with dementia typically manifests first with parkinsonian symptoms, whereas LBD manifests first with dementia. Resting tremor is a common feature of Parkinson disease that is rarely seen in LBD.

Delirium is characterized by an acute disturbance in attention with a waxing and waning of symptoms that may include hallucinations. It is not necessarily associated with dementia or parkinsonism.

Pathogenesis

LBD shares characteristics with both Parkinson disease and Alzheimer disease but is a unique diagnostic entity. LBD features **Lewy bodies** and **deficits in dopaminergic function** (as in Parkinson disease) as well as **senile plaques** and **deficits in cholinergic function** (as in Alzheimer disease). Clinically, LBD presents with characteristic clinical features of **chronic cognitive decline, visual hallucinations,** and **parkinsonian symptoms of bradykinesia and rigidity** (resting tremor is rarely seen). The cognitive decline seen in LBD has a chronic course, although it **may fluctuate throughout the course of the day** in a pattern similar to the waxing and waning of delirium.

Management

As with Alzheimer dementia, **cholinesterase inhibitors** (donepezil, rivastigmine) can be used to slow the progression of cognitive decline. **Dopamine agonists** may be used to treat parkinsonian symptoms, although these medications can exacerbate visual hallucinations. **Typical neuroleptics should be completely avoided,** and atypical neuroleptics should be used sparingly for agitation and hallucinations because these medications can exacerbate parkinsonism and increase mortality. Nonpharmacologic treatment should focus on care-giver education and support, as well as on reconfiguration of the home environment to maximize safety.

Breakout Point

Charles Bonnet syndrome describes the common occurrence of visual hallucinations in the visually impaired. This syndrome differs from LBD in that the patient with Charles Bonnet syndrome has good insight that they are seeing things that are not actually there.

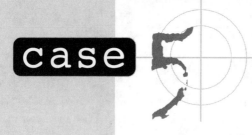

case 5

CC A 19-year-old male college student with **unusual facial movements** presents to his student health center, noting that he accidentally left his medication at home.

HPI The patient reports that he began having embarrassing problems with **blinking** at the age of 7 years. Over the next few years, he developed an impulse to repeatedly glance sideways, and he began **snorting** and **grunting**. The patient says that his most bothersome symptom "is when my right arm jerks up. I pretend like I am just scratching the back of my neck or sometimes I leave it raised in class, like I have a question."

PE Prominent repeated **eye-blinking, nose-scrunching,** and scratching of his neck.

Labs Not relevant.

Imaging Not relevant.

case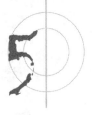

Tourette Disorder

Differential

Transient tic disorder is diagnosed in patients younger than 18 years of age and features motor and/or vocal tics occurring for at least 4 weeks but resolving within 12 months.

Pervasive developmental disorders often feature stereotypical behaviors such as hand wringing, rocking, and flapping. These are usually associated with marked deficits in different cognitive domains.

Movement disorders (eg, Huntington disease, Wilson disease) include a variety of involuntary movements. These typically have a later onset and are associated with other physical or laboratory findings.

Pathogenesis

Tourette disorder is a tic disorder involving **multiple motor tics** and **one or more vocal tics,** with an **onset before 18 years of age.** Initial symptoms include tics of the face and neck, with progression to other muscle groups and vocal tics. Common simple vocal tics include coughing, throat clearing, and snorting. More complex vocal and motor tics can also occur. Genetic factors play a role in the illness, with sons of affected mothers at greatest risk for developing it.

Epidemiology

It is two to three times **more common in boys** and typically begins by age 7 in boys and age 11 in girls. Up to 50% of patients with Tourette disorder suffer comorbid ADHD and about 40% have OCD.

Management

Treatment involves parental and teacher education that tics are involuntary. Behavior therapy aimed at self-monitoring and teaching patients "counter" movements used to thwart a tic or turn it into a socially acceptable motion (such as head scratching) can be helpful. Neuroleptics (haloperidol, pimozide) can reduce tics significantly, but problematic adverse effects limit their use. Any comorbid disorders (particularly ADHD and OCD) should be addressed; however, the **stimulant medications used to treat ADHD may worsen tics.**

Breakout Point

> Coprolalia (the repeated utterance of obscene words) is a feature of Tourette disorder often highlighted in the media but occurring in only 15% of patients.

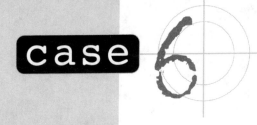

CC   A 44-year-old man is admitted to the trauma service after falling down a flight of stairs. A psychiatry consult is requested after the patient endorsed "**hearing voices.**"

HPI   The patient reports increasingly frequent **episodes of hearing strange voices** over the past few months. He believes his symptoms started **after he was struck on the head** at work. Prior to each episode, he reports a **strange rising sensation in his chest and abdomen.** He endorses a similar sensation prior to his fall but is unable to recall other details of the event.

PE   Multiple orthopedic injuries; otherwise normal physical and neurological exam.

Labs   Toxicology screens: negative.

case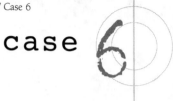

Complex Partial Seizures (CPS)

Differential

Psychosis as a result of psychiatric illness may present with hallucinations and odd behavior. Careful history and EEG studies are important to accurate diagnosis.

Delirium can present with waxing and waning cognition associated with hallucinations. Again, careful history and EEG studies are important to accurate diagnosis. EEG in delirium due to a general medical condition typically reveals generalized theta-delta slowing, whereas EEG in delirium due to alcohol or sedative-hypnotics usually shows rapid beta activity.

Pathogenesis

CPS of the temporal lobe, also referred to as temporal lobe epilepsy (TLE) or limbic epilepsy, can present with a wide variety of symptoms, many of which may mimic primary psychiatric illness. Psychotic symptoms, including hallucinations, are estimated to occur in 10% of patients with CPS. Other common symptoms include **motor automatisms** and **staring spells.** A rising sensation in the chest and/or abdomen has been classically described as an aura associated with this phenomenon. CPS often initiate around a seizure focus that may be the result of mechanical injury, neoplasm, or stroke. Partial seizure activity can progress to generalized tonic-clonic seizure activity, as may have happened in this case precipitating the patient's fall. Due to their bizarre presentations and absence of tonic-clonic motor activity, **patients with CPS are often misdiagnosed with psychiatric illnesses.** EEG, especially between episodes, may be equivocal because the seizure activity may be occurring in deep structures far removed from the scalp.

Management

As with other seizure disorders, CPS should be treated with anticonvulsant medications (valproate, phenytoin, carbamazepine, oxcarbazepine). IV benzodiazepines may help "break" active seizure activity.

Breakout Point

> The existence of an interictal personality type for patients with TLE (consisting of religiosity, hypergraphia, and "viscosity of personality") is controversial.

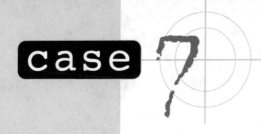

case 7

CC A 42-year-old woman is referred to a psychiatrist for **depressed mood** after having been **fired from her job** 3 months ago.

HPI Since her dismissal, she has become **withdrawn** and is **overwhelmed** by the thought that no one will hire her. Her **symptoms seem out of proportion to the stress** of having lost her job. On careful screening, she **does not fulfill the criteria for a major depressive episode.**

PE Physical and neurologic exams are within normal limits.

case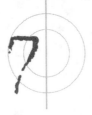

Adjustment Disorder

Differential

Major depressive disorder is distinguished from adjustment disorder because adjustment disorder does not fulfill five of the nine criteria for major depressive disorder (depressed mood; anhedonia; decreased energy/fatigue; sleep disturbance; appetite change; psychomotor retardation or agitation; feelings of excessive guilt and/or hopelessness; decreased concentration/memory; and morbid preoccupations, including suicidality). In diagnosing adjustment disorder, there must be an identifiable stressor within the 3 months prior to the occurrence of symptoms.

Anxiety disorders (generalized anxiety disorder, panic disorder, PTSD) can be distinguished from adjustment disorder on the basis of symptom quality and severity. Flashbacks, hyperarousal states, and panic attacks generally do not occur in adjustment disorder. The typical initial stressor of PTSD is a trauma of unusual or catastrophic character.

Pathogenesis

Adjustment disorder is prompted by an **identifiable stressor** (occurring within the 3 months prior to the occurrence of symptoms) that arises against a backdrop of biological and psychosocial factors. Once the stressor and its consequences have terminated, the symptoms do not persist for more than 6 months. Subtypes of adjustment disorder are identified by the presence of depressed mood, anxiety, disturbance of conduct, or combinations of these symptoms.

Epidemiology

These disorders are about **twice as common in women** than in men.

Management

Short-term **psychotherapy**, to identify the stressors and develop new approaches to coping, is the treatment of choice. If the patient is refractory to psychotherapy, or if depressed/anxious symptoms are prominent, pharmacotherapy should be considered. **Benzodiazepines** (lorazepam, clonazepam, alprazolam) are useful for controlling anxiety, whereas **antidepressants** may be helpful for depressive symptoms.

Breakout Point

Common Stressors That Can Precipitate Adjustment Disorders
End of a Relationship
Financial Difficulties
Diagnosis with a Medical Illness
Geographic Changes (eg, going away to college)
Retirement
Death of a loved one is not included because bereavement is considered a separate diagnostic entity.

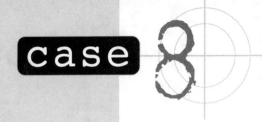

case 8

CC A 32-year-old woman seeks help because she fears she is going to lose her job.

HPI She works for a large firm in the financial district and was recently promoted. Her promotion has taken her from an office on the 9th floor to an office on the 32nd floor of the building. She reports a long-standing inability to ride on elevators due to **overwhelming fear** accompanied by **palpitations, diaphoresis,** and **dyspnea.** She has always taken the stairs to her office, but now this has made her late for numerous meetings, drawing the attention of her supervisor. She realizes that her fear is irrational but has been unable to change her behavior. She reports normal sleep, appetite, and energy levels. There is no past history of traumatic events or obsessive-compulsive behavior.

PE Physical and neurologic exam normal.

Labs Lytes/CBC: normal. TFTs: normal. UA: toxicology negative.

Imaging Not relevant.

case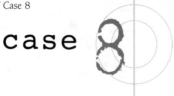

Specific Phobia

Differential

Panic disorder with agoraphobia describes panic attacks accompanied by a fear that they will occur in places where escape would be difficult or help may not be available.

Social phobia should be diagnosed if the fear of embarrassment and anxiety are directly related to social- or performance-related situations.

Pathogenesis

Phobias are thought to result from unconscious conditioning of a fearful response to a **specific stimulus.** In some cases (spiders, snakes), phobic responses may represent an adaptive evolutionary response.

Epidemiology

Approximately 10% of the population meets criteria for diagnosis with a specific phobia. The condition is more common in women than in men, and onset typically occurs in childhood or adolescence.

Management

CBT is at least as effective as pharmacotherapy. Commonly used techniques include **systemic desensitization** (repeated, gradually increasing exposure to the stimulus), and **flooding** (precipitous and sustained exposure until the response subsides). **Benzodiazepines** are also effective and provide rapid symptomatic relief in the acute period. **Propranolol** may be used if sympathetic hyperarousal is prominent.

Breakout Point

Some of the Most Common Specific Phobias:
Claustrophobia: Fear of Enclosed Spaces
Aviatophobia: Fear of Flying
Acrophobia: Fear of Heights
Hemophobia: Fear of Blood
Trypanophobia: Fear of Injections
Arachnophobia: Fear of Spiders
Ophidiophobia: Fear of Snakes
Astraphobia: Fear of Thunderstorms

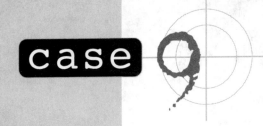

case 9

CC A 29-year-old married **woman** visits her internist because she has been unable to conceive for 3 months.

HPI The patient is **restless and fidgety,** stating that she is worried that she might not be able to have a child. After being offered reassurance, she indicates that she has felt **on edge** for **at least the past 6 months.** She also admits to being **irritable** and adds that she has had **trouble falling asleep.** She constantly **worries most of the day** about various things, such as whether her husband will leave her, whether something might happen to her mother, and whether her boss will fire her. She states that her worries create **muscle tension** and **impaired concentration.**

PE Physical and neurologic exam normal.

Labs Lytes/CBC: normal. TFTs: normal. UA: toxicology screen negative. ECG: normal.

Imaging Not relevant.

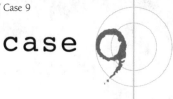

case 9

Generalized Anxiety Disorder (GAD)

Differential

Anxiety disorder due to a general medical condition is diagnosed if a patient has a medical condition that results in anxiety.

Panic disorder is characterized by spontaneous episodes of panic followed by a debilitating fear of recurrent attacks.

Substance-induced anxiety disorder may be precipitated by caffeine, cocaine, thyroxine, alcohol, theophylline, and corticosteroids.

Hypochondriasis presents with anxiety that is related to the specific fear of having an illness.

Pathogenesis

GAD has been associated with various neurotransmitters, although it is likely that an interaction between biological and psychosocial factors lead to the disorder. GAD is a very common condition that is frequently seen in primary care.

Management

Psychotherapy, relaxation techniques, and lifestyle modification (reduction of caffeine or other stimulants) are useful **psychosocial interventions.** Pharmacologic agents used to treat GAD include **benzodiazepines, TCAs** (clomipramine), **SSRIs,** or atypical antidepressants such as serotonin-norepinephrine reuptake inhibitors (venlafaxine, duloxetine). Symptoms may not improve until SSRIs and other antidepressants have been used for 1 to 4 weeks. Administration of benzodiazepines in the acute period can provide the patient with rapid symptomatic relief while waiting for the antidepressants to take effect. **Beta-blockers** (propranolol) or **alpha-adrenergic antagonists** (clonidine) can be helpful in diminishing excess sympathetic outflow (to relieve palpitations, increased HR, and tremor), although typically they are not effective for the full range of anxiety symptoms seen in GAD.

Breakout Point

Symptoms of Generalized Anxiety Disorder (WATCHERS)	
Worry	**H**yperarousal
Anxiety	**E**nergy Loss
Tension	**R**estlessness
Concentration Problems	**S**leep Problems

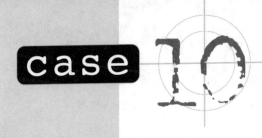

case 10

CC A 28-year-old man presents to the ER worried that his chapped hands may have become infected.

HPI The patient has been **obsessed** with thoughts of infection and spends **several hours each day scrubbing his hands.** His persistent and **intrusive thoughts** regarding infections are quite **distressing** (ego dystonic), making it difficult for him to leave his home. The patient also admits to being afraid that he will accidentally leave his stove on (obsessions), and he **checks his stove exactly 29 times** before leaving the house or going to bed (compulsions). The patient **acknowledges that his behavior is senseless** but is unable to control it.

PE Severely desquamated skin with mild bleeding over both hands.

Labs Not relevant.

Imaging Not relevant.

case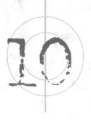

Obsessive-Compulsive Disorder (OCD)

Differential

Obsessive-compulsive personality disorder (OCPD) is associated with chronic, pervasive personality traits such as rigidity, perfectionism, and orderliness; it lacks the true obsessions and compulsions present in OCD. Patients with OCPD do not feel that their actions are inconsistent with their overall personality, whereas patients with OCD report that their actions are foreign and distressing.

Anxiety disorders can be distinguished from OCD by their lack of specific rituals, obsessions, and compulsions.

Pathogenesis

Genetic and neurobiologic factors have been implicated in the pathogenesis of OCD. Structural and neurochemical abnormalities located in the orbitofrontal cortex and basal ganglia have been associated with OCD.

Epidemiology

Lifetime prevalence of OCD is 2% to 3%; males and females are affected in equal number. Childhood-onset OCD is more common in males and more likely to be related to ADHD and Tourette syndrome.

Management

First-line medication includes **high-dose SSRIs** and the TCA **clomipramine** over a period of 16 to 18 weeks. **Behavioral therapy,** involving evoking obsessions and preventing subsequent compulsive behaviors (eg, touching a "dirty" doorknob, then preventing hand washing), is important in the treatment of OCD. In extreme cases of refractory OCD, neurosurgery (cingulotomy, limbic leucotomy, or anterior capsulotomy) may be useful.

Breakout Point

> Sudden onset of OCD in children has been associated with GABHS infection. The syndrome is known as **pediatric autoimmune neuropsychiatric disorders associated with streptococcal infection (PANDAS).**

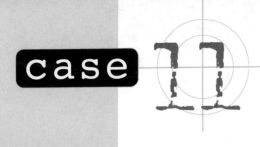

case 11

CC A 35-year-old **woman** presents to a cardiologist after recurrent episodes of **chest pain, palpitations,** and **dizziness.**

HPI The patient's symptoms arose while she was on a bus going to work, lasting for **less than 10 minutes.** She was unable to identify any specific trigger for that initial episode. She had two more similar episodes that were sufficiently intense that she **thought she was going to die** (feelings of impending doom). Since these episodes, she **fears recurrent attacks** and **experiences anxiety when she has to leave the house.** Other symptoms that occur during the attacks include **nausea, sweating, tingling sensations** (paresthesias), and **hot flashes.**

PE Physical and neurologic exam normal.

Labs Lytes/CBC: normal. Vitamin B_{12} and folate: normal; TFTs within normal limits; RPR/VDRL nonreactive. UA: normal; urine toxicology negative; urinary catecholamines normal. ECG: normal sinus rhythm with no evidence of ischemia or infarction.

Imaging Not relevant.

case 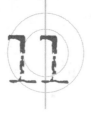 11

Panic Disorder

Differential

Anxiety disorder due to general medical condition is diagnosed if a patient has a medical condition that results in anxiety. Substance-induced anxiety disorder may be precipitated by caffeine, cocaine, thyroxine, alcohol, theophylline, and corticosteroids. Hypochondriasis presents with anxiety that is related to the specific fear of having an illness.

PTSD involves panic attacks related to specific traumatic stimuli or cues.

Agoraphobia is the fear of being in places or situations from which it might be difficult or embarrassing to escape in the event of a panic attack. Panic attacks can occur with or without the development of agoraphobia.

Pathogenesis

Panic disorder has been linked to dysregulation of both central and peripheral (autonomic) nervous systems.

Epidemiology

Prevalence is 1% to 3%, with **females** affected **more often than males** by a ratio of 2 to 1.

Management

Psychotherapy, relaxation techniques, and lifestyle modification (reduction of caffeine or other stimulant drugs) are useful psychosocial interventions. **CBT** has been shown to be as, or more, effective than pharmacotherapy in the long-term treatment of panic disorder. Pharmacologic agents used to treat GAD include **benzodiazepines, TCAs** (clomipramine), **SSRIs,** serotonin-norepinephrine reuptake inhibitors (venlafaxine, duloxetine), and MAO inhibitors (phenelzine).

Symptom improvement may not occur until SSRIs and other antidepressants have been taken for 1 to 4 weeks. Administration of benzodiazepines in the acute period can provide the patient with rapid symptomatic relief while waiting for the therapeutic effect of the SSRIs, TCAs, or buspirone to take effect. **Beta-blockers** (propranolol) or **alpha-adrenergic antagonists** (clonidine) can be helpful in diminishing excess sympathetic outflow (to relieve palpitations, increased HR, and tremor), but these drugs are not effective for the full range of anxiety symptoms seen in panic disorder, so are best used as an adjunct.

Breakout Point

Medical Conditions That May Present with Anxiety: Physical Diseases That Have Commonly Appeared Anxious	
Pheochromocytoma	Carcinoid
Diabetes Mellitus	Alcohol Withdrawal
Temporal Lobe Epilepsy	Arrhythmias
Hyperthyroidism	

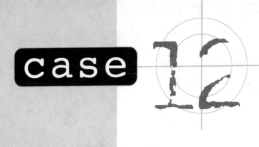

case 12

CC   A 21-year-old **woman** college student presents to her primary care physician complaining of **irritability, anxiety, trouble sleeping,** and **difficulty concentrating.**

HPI   She reports feeling more **withdrawn** from friends over the past few months and is now starting to miss classes. She says she is **fearful** of walking through Harvard Square, frequently **avoiding** it altogether, and expresses doubt about whether she will be able to complete her studies. She reveals that 6 months ago she was **raped** by a male acquaintance while walking across campus. She describes feeling **intense helplessness** and **horror** during the event. For **more than 1 month,** she has been experiencing horrible **nightmares** and **flashbacks** of being sexually assaulted.

PE   Patient **hypervigilant** throughout exam and demonstrates an **exaggerated startle reaction.**

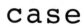

case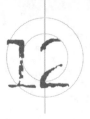

Post-Traumatic Stress Disorder (PTSD)

Differential

Acute stress disorder is diagnosed when symptoms occur within 1 month of the stressor and symptoms do not last more than 1 month. A diagnosis of acute stress disorder progresses to a diagnosis of PTSD if the symptoms persist for more than 1 month.

Major depression involves symptoms, such as anhedonia, restricted affect, poor concentration, and feelings of detachment, but recurrent and intrusive trauma-related recollections and hypervigilance are not present.

Panic disorder and **GAD** may present with autonomic hyperactivity but lack the specific inciting traumatic event of PTSD.

OCD and PTSD both involve repetitive and intrusive symptoms; if the symptoms can be linked to a traumatic origin, PTSD is the likely diagnosis.

Adjustment disorder represents a brief maladaptive response to life stressors that is not associated with the constellation of symptoms seen in PTSD.

Pathogenesis

PTSD is defined by its causative origin—there must be a **severe identifiable stressor** that results in its distressing symptomatology. A latency period of months to years may intervene between the trauma and the onset of symptoms. Symptoms present with a triad of **re-experience** (nightmares, flashbacks), **avoidance,** and **increased arousal** (hypervigilance, poor concentration, insomnia). Increased rates of PTSD are seen in groups that have experienced severe trauma (eg, survivors of natural disaster, war veterans).

Management

Psychotherapy is key to long-term recovery. Pharmacotherapy is used to target prominent symptoms such as depression, anxiety, or intrusive thoughts. Drugs found helpful include **SSRIs, TCAs,** and **MAO inhibitors.** Benzodiazepines, beta-blockers, and alpha adrenergic antagonists (clonidine) may be useful to counter hyperarousal.

Breakout Point

Clinical Presentation of PTSD (TRAUMA)
Traumatic Event
Re-experience
Avoidance
Unable to Function
Month Long or More Duration of Symptoms
Arousal Is Increased

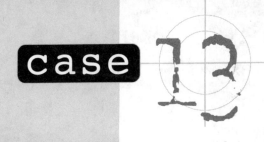

case 13

CC A 23-year-old **woman** graduate student experiences **intense anxiety** at research meetings when she is asked to contribute her comments. She also has **excessive fears that she will act in a manner that will be embarrassing** at social events.

HPI Her anxiety is accompanied by **sweating, trembling,** and **palpitations** during these meetings. She is **concerned that she will embarrass herself,** although she **realizes that her anxiety is excessive for the situation.** She experiences similar symptoms in other performance situations and at social gatherings.

PE Physical and neurologic exam normal.

Labs Lytes/CBC: normal. Vitamin B_{12} and folate: normal; TFTs: normal; RPR/VDRL nonreactive. UA: normal; toxicology negative.

ANXIETY DISORDER

case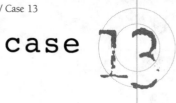

Social Phobia

Differential

Separation anxiety disorder is seen in children who are reluctant to enter social situations out of a concern for leaving their care-taker; however, they are comfortable in social situations with their caretaker present.

Avoidant personality disorder describes a maladaptive and per-vasive personality pattern involving an avoidance of interpersonal contact for fear of being rejected and a preoccupation with being criticized or feeling inadequate. This diagnosis may coexist with generalized social phobia and may be clinically indistinguishable from social phobias.

Specific phobia involves anxiety related to a specific object or situ-ation that does not involve scrutiny, humiliation, or embarrassment. Exposure to the feared stimulus provokes an immediate response.

Panic disorder with agoraphobia describes panic attacks with a fear of places in which escape would be difficult or a fear that help may not be available if needed. These attacks are not limited to social situations.

Pathogenesis

Social phobia (or social anxiety disorder) is marked by a **persist-ent fear of embarrassment or scrutiny in group settings.** The etiology of social phobia is unknown, but genetic, learning, per-sonality, and biologic factors have been implicated.

Epidemiology

Lifetime prevalence is 3% to 13%; onset typically occurs in **adoles-cence.**

Management

SSRIs, serotonin-norepinephrine reuptake inhibitors (venlafaxine, duloxetine), or TCAs can reduce symptoms of anxiety. **Beta-blockers** limit sympathetic outflow and can be taken prophylactically before stress-inducing events such as presentations or social gatherings. Benzodiazepines may useful in the short-term. **CBT** is effective and includes relaxation strategies, social skills development, cognitive retraining, and desensitization.

Breakout Point

Diagnostic Criteria of Social Phobia (FAINT)

Fear of Social or Performance Situations
Anxiety When Exposed to the **S**ituations/**A**voidance of the Situations
Insight into the Unreasonableness of the Fear/Interference with Functioning
Not Due to Medication or a Medical Condition
Timing: In Patients under 18 Years of Age, Symptoms Persist for at Least 6 Months

case 14

CC   A 9-year-old **boy** is brought to the pediatrician's office with **difficulty organizing tasks, trouble following instructions, forgetting homework assignments,** and **losing things.**

HPI He also **makes careless mistakes** in his schoolwork and often **does not seem to listen when spoken to directly.** According to his parents, the patient has always been forgetful and inattentive, but his problems have worsened over the past 6 months and resulting in **poor grades.** Teachers report that he **fidgets** at his desk and **talks more** than other students. Classmates become angry with him because he interrupts and impulsively **blurts out answers.** He often leaves his seat in the classroom and runs around excessively at recess.

PE   Young boy unable to sit still in chair and rapidly tapping feet together; physical and neurologic exams normal.

Labs CBC, Lytes, TFTs, and lead level all within normal limits.

case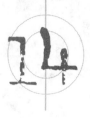

Attention-Deficit Hyperactivity Disorder (ADHD)

Differential

Conduct disorder is marked by violations of the basic rights of others or of age-appropriate societal norms. If conduct disorder exists without comorbid ADHD, attention and cognitive organization should be normal.

Major depressive disorder may mimic ADHD with symptoms of inattention, cognitive dysfunction, and irritability. Careful history should include evaluation for mood changes, neurovegetative symptoms, and suicidality.

Pervasive developmental and learning disorders must also be distinguished from ADHD, but it should be noted that ADHD frequently coexists with learning disorders.

Pathogenesis

No specific cause of ADHD has been identified; a combination of genetic, neurobiologic, environmental (perinatal/neonatal trauma), and psychosocial factors have been implicated. For a diagnosis of ADHD, some **symptoms of hyperactivity-impulsivity or inattention must have been present before the age of 7 years**, and impairment must be present **in two or more settings** (eg, at home and at school). Risk factors include family history of ADHD, family discord, low birth weight, and early brain insults. It has been estimated that approximately 70% of children diagnosed with ADHD continue to have symptoms into adolescence (contrary to the myth that children "outgrow" ADHD). Without treatment, patients are at increased risk for substance abuse later in life. **Males are diagnosed more often than females,** but this may be due to boys presenting more frequently with disruptive hyperactivity rather than quiet inattention.

Management

Treatments include **pharmacologic intervention** and **behavioral therapy. Stimulants** such as **methylphenidate** (Ritalin) or amphetamine salts (Adderall) are the most established pharmacologic treatments. **Atomoxetine** (Strattera, a selective norepinephrine reuptake inhibitor) is a newer medication with a specific indication for ADHD. Patients receiving stimulant therapy may develop **vocal or motor tics,** weight loss, insomnia, and tremor.

Breakout Point

> It is important to check a lead level in children with learning or behavioral difficulties, because lead poisoning (usually due to lead-containing paint in older houses) can present with a variety of neuropsychiatric symptoms.

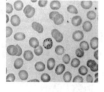

Figure 14-1. Hypochromia and basophilic stippling of erythrocytes seen in lead poisoning.

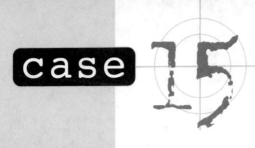

case 15

CC   A 4-year-old **boy** is brought to his pediatrician by his parents, concerned with their son's **difficulty playing with other children** at preschool.

HPI   **Before the age of 3 years** he had been evaluated numerous times for **speech delay** and **odd behaviors**. He has continued to have difficulties, and his new preschool teacher has commented on his preference to play alone at recess. His **eye contact is poor**, and his **facial expression emotionless**. He often repeats what other people say, and his parents report that he **does not seek interaction with others**, appearing to be interested only in examining his toy cars.

PE   Blank facial expression; does not engage in conversation; behavior notable for **stereotyped movements** of **rocking** and **hand flapping**; rather than playing with toys, patient arranges them in lines; IQ 75; normal physical characteristics and neurologic exam.

Labs   Lytes/CBC: normal. TFTs: normal; heavy metal panel negative; hearing test shows no abnormality; chromosomal analysis negative for fragile X syndrome. EEG: no abnormality.

Imaging Not relevant.

case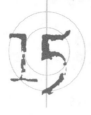

Autism

Differential

Asperger syndrome describes social impairments similar to autism without significant impairment in language or IQ.

Rett syndrome involves **deceleration of head growth,** stereotyped hand wringing movements, poorly coordinated gait, and impairment in language, occurring **only in girls** between the ages of 5 months and $2\frac{1}{2}$ years.

Mental retardation is diagnosed when **IQ is less than 70;** it often coexists with autism.

Psychosocial deprivation can result in autism-like symptoms but may improve when the environment is corrected.

Medical conditions may present with autistic symptoms; these include fragile X syndrome, Down syndrome, tuberous sclerosis, and phenylketonuria. A thorough medical workup is critical.

Pathogenesis

Autism is a pervasive developmental disorder incorporating **impairments in social interaction, impairments in communication, and repetitive and stereotyped behaviors, interests, and activities,** with **onset of symptoms before 3 years of age.** No specific cause for autism has been identified, but neuroanatomical, infectious, genetic, and perinatal insults have been implicated. About 75% of children with autism are also diagnosed with mental retardation. Only 1% to 2% of patients achieve normal independent status in adulthood. Predictors of better prognosis include higher IQ, better language skills, and later age of onset.

Epidemiology

Prevalence is 0.05%, with **males affected more often than females** by a ratio of 4 to 1.

Management

Psychoeducation and support for parents is vital. Intense and structured academic and language remediation is often required. **Behavioral therapy** is used to reinforce normal social behaviors. Medications can provide symptomatic relief. **Neuroleptics** may reduce hyperactivity and aggression, and **SSRIs** are used to treat obsessive-compulsive features and stereotypical behaviors.

Breakout Point

> Despite claims in the popular media, research has produced no significant evidence linking autism to the MMR vaccine.

CC   A 10-year-old **girl** is brought to the pediatrician's office as a follow-up visit for pharyngitis.

HPI   Two weeks earlier, the pediatrician had recommended fluid and bed rest, but since then, the patient has complained of worsening sore throat, difficulty swallowing, and abdominal pain. The mother notes that her daughter has been anxious, irritable, and "not acting herself."

PE   Significant for erythema of the posterior oropharynx with grayish exudate; abdominal exam normal; neurologic exam normal.

Labs   Lytes/CBC: normal. Throat culture grows *Neisseria gonorrhoeae* on chocolate agar and Thayer-Martin medium.

case 16

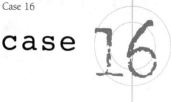

Child Sexual Abuse

Differential

Physical abuse is characterized by signs such as cuts or bruises in low-trauma areas (buttocks, genitals, back), burns to the perineum or burns with suspicious patterns (immersion scalding, cigarette marks), multiple fractures of different ages, **spiral fractures of long bones,** and **retinal hemorrhages** ("shaken baby syndrome"). In contrast to sexual abuse, perpetrators of physical abuse of children are most often female.

Neglect may present with malnutrition, poor hygiene, delayed developmental milestones, and failure to thrive. Neglected children are frequently indiscriminately affectionate with strangers.

Pathogenesis

The perpetrator of sexual abuse of a child is often someone known to the victim, usually a trusted **male** family member or friend. There are no specific behaviors that definitively indicate the experience of sexual abuse, but **sexualized play, aggression,** and **withdrawal** are all frequently seen in victims.

Epidemiology

One in every four girls and one in every eight boys suffers some form of sexual assault before the age of 18 years.

Management

Steps should be taken to **ensure the safety of not only the patient, but of all the children in the home. Reporting to child protective services** whenever there is even suspicion of any form of child abuse is **mandated by law.** Once the existence of abuse has been confirmed, individual psychotherapy can begin to address the long-term sequelae of abuse. Sexual abuse as a child has been implicated in the development of **adult psychiatric disorders** such as major depressive disorder, substance abuse, borderline personality disorder, PTSD, and dissociative disorders.

Breakout Point

> Interview of a child regarding abuse (even superficially simple questions such as "Did he touch you here?") should always be deferred to a specialist in order to avoid "leading the witness" and ensure admissibility of the information obtained for any future legal proceedings brought against the abuser.

CC A **13-year-old boy** is referred to the child psychiatry clinic for **repeatedly starting fights** and **stealing**.

HPI School records reveal increasingly out-of-control behavior for **at least the past 6 months**. The patient has **run away from home** several times, often **stays out late despite curfews,** and frequently **misses classes.** He has been arrested for vandalism, which has included **setting fires.** When interviewed, the patient **denies any wrongdoing.**

PE On interview, the patient is uncooperative, hostile, and provocative.

case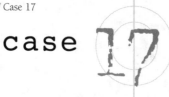

Conduct Disorder

Differential

Oppositional defiant disorder is distinguished by predominantly negativistic, defiant, and hostile behaviors without serious violations of social norms or the rights of others.

Depressive disorders in children and adolescents often present with agitation, irritability, and disruptive behavior. Careful history and assessment of mood can help differentiate depression from conduct disorder.

Substance abuse disorders may produce manifestations of conduct disorder. Careful history and urine toxicology screens are important for an accurate diagnosis.

Antisocial personality disorder cannot be diagnosed in an individual younger than 18 years of age.

Pathogenesis

Conduct disorder presents with a consistent pattern of violation of the rights of others or of major societal rules, frequently including behaviors of aggression, destruction of property, deceit, and theft. Risk factors include **parental divorce, chaotic home environments, negligence, parental psychopathology,** and **harshly punitive parental style.** Physiologically, there is some evidence of decreased levels of noradrenergic functioning and of decreased serotonin metabolites in the CSF.

Epidemiology

Male:female ratio is 4:1. Comorbidity with **ADHD** and substance abuse is high.

Management

Multimodal treatment programs mobilizing community and family resources and a **firm environmental structure** with consistent rules and expected consequences form the cornerstone of treatment. A number of **medications may be useful in the treatment of associated symptoms.** Carbamazepine, clonidine, lithium, and propranolol have all been used to treat impulsive aggression. **Treatment of comorbid disorders** (ADHD, depression, substance abuse syndromes, and learning disorders) may help further ameliorate symptomatology. Conduct disorder in childhood may progress to a diagnosis of **antisocial personality disorder** as an adult. Both have been classically associated with a triad of enuresis, cruelty to animals, and fire-setting.

Breakout Point

Remember:

Conduct Disorder is a Diagnosis of **C**hildren
Antisocial Personality Disorder is a Diagnosis of **A**dults

CC   A **6-year-old girl** is brought to her pediatrician's office after several episodes of **screaming at night.**

HPI   According to her parents, shortly after falling asleep, the patient sits up in bed **crying** and **appearing frightened** while **breathing rapidly and sweating.** The episodes **last no more than 10 minutes,** during which she is **not responsive to comforting comments.** The patient is **unable to recall any details** of these experiences.

PE   Physical and neurologic exams normal.

case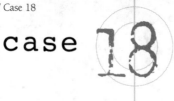

Sleep Terror Disorder

Differential

Nightmare disorder occurs in the second half of the night during REM sleep, and the individual has vivid recollections of the dream.

Sleepwalking disorder has a greater degree of organized motor activity, occurs in stages III and IV of non-REM sleep and is not remembered the next morning. Sleepwalking disorder and sleep terrors often coexist.

Seizure disorders may present with stereotyped behavior and postictal confusion; EEG may help identify seizure disorders.

Panic disorder may cause patients to awaken at night in a state of fear and hyperarousal; however, the motor hyperactivity and amnesia characteristic of sleep terror are not seen.

Pathogenesis

Sleep terror disorder is **arousal during the first third of the night, occurring during stages III and IV of non-REM sleep.** It is usually heralded by a scream or cry, followed by the physiologic manifestations of extreme anxiety. Patients typically return to sleep within 10 minutes and have no memory of the episode. Sleep terror disorder occurs in 1% to 6% of children, and tends to run in families. Age of onset is between 4 and 12 years of age in children, and the condition **usually resolves spontaneously** by early adolescence.

Management

The patient and family should be reassured that the behavior is usually outgrown by adolescence. Safety measures are important to protect the individual from injury. The individual **should not be deliberately awakened** during an episode of sleep terror or sleepwalking, because this may exacerbate confusion and terror. Pharmacologic management is typically unnecessary, because the behavior often resolves on its own, but if sleep terrors are severe, pharmacologic management with **benzodiazepines** or **imipramine** may prove useful.

Breakout Point

> Hypnagogic and hypnopompic hallucinations occur during the stages of falling asleep and waking up, respectively. Remember: Hypna**GO**gic hallucinations occur while **GO**ing to sleep.

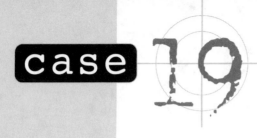

case 19

CC A 3-year-old boy presents to the pediatric clinic; his mother is concerned about his chronic **constipation and fatigue.**

HPI Further questioning reveals that the child has a poor diet and has been seen **ingesting paint chips** from the wall of their apartment. The mother is raising this child as well as four other children by herself and often works long hours, leaving the older children to watch the 3-year-old. **Supervision** of the child during these times is questionable.

PE **Deceleration noted on growth curve.**

Labs **Iron deficiency anemia; basophilic stippling of erythrocytes; serum lead levels >10 μg/dL.**

Imaging

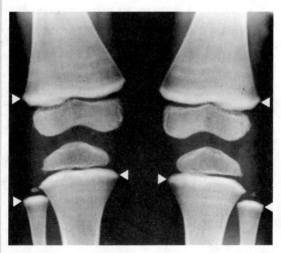

Figure 19-1. Dense transverse bands extending across the metaphyses of long bones.

case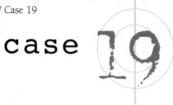

Pica

Differential

Pica is often associated with other comorbid conditions, including schizophrenia, mental retardation, pregnancy, autism, dementia, and delirium.

Pathogenesis

Pica involves the **repeated consumption of nonfood substances over the course of at least 1 month.** It most commonly occurs in toddlers, pregnant women, and mentally retarded adults. Low socioeconomic status, environmental deprivation, parental psychopathology, nutritional deficiencies, iron deficiency anemia, and boredom are risk factors.

Management

Consumption of some nonfood substances can be relatively harmless, but the patient should receive **behavioral therapy** (and the parents should receive appropriate education and guidance) to encourage proper nutrition. Consumption of paint chips in older houses poses risk of significant morbidity due to lead poisoning. **Lead poisoning** can present with stunted growth, reduced IQ, discoloration of the gingiva ("lead lines"), and deposition in the metaphyses of long bones. If lead levels are greater than 10 μg/dL, chelation therapy may be indicated. **Iron deficiency anemia** should be corrected with iron supplementation.

Breakout Point

> Lead-based paints were banned for residential use in the United States in 1978.

case 20

CC A 9-year-old boy is referred to the child psychiatry clinic due to **frequent teasing** at school.

HPI The patient's mother reports that he has always had **difficulty making and maintaining friends due to poor social skills.** His **interests differ from those of his peers** and are **more narrowly focused.** For example, whereas his classmates are interested in various cartoon characters, sports, and hobbies, he is fascinated by dinosaurs and has an extensive collection of dinosaur models, books, and movies. His interest in dinosaurs seems to preclude any other hobbies or pursuits. He tends to **lecture adults and peers** in a monotonic voice about dinosaurs and does not notice when people become bored or disinterested. He does **well academically** and has no learning issues. His **use of language is good,** and other than **minor delays in motor development,** his developmental history is unremarkable.

case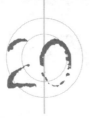

Asperger Disorder

Differential

Rett syndrome involves **deceleration of head growth**, stereotyped hand wringing movements, poorly coordinated gait, and impairment in language, occurring **only in girls** between 5 months and $2^1/_2$ years of age.

Autism is characterized by marked impairment in social interaction, language development, and stereotyped patterns of behavior.

Asperger disorder is not associated with deficits in language.

Childhood disintegrative disorder is characterized by a developmental regression and loss of previously acquired language, social, or motor skills occurring after 2 years of age.

Pathogenesis

Asperger disorder is characterized by significant **impairment in social interaction** and **restricted, repetitive, and stereotyped patterns of behavior and interests** without delays in language or cognition. Patients with the diagnosis often exhibit difficulty in reading nonverbal social cues and in the employment of nonverbal communication (eye contact, facial expression, body posture). This, combined with their focused and idiosyncratic interests, can lead to difficulty with social integration.

Management

Management of Asperger disorder includes teaching of **pragmatic language skills** and **social skills groups** with peers.

Breakout Point

> Some patients with Asperger disorder or autism present with remarkable aptitude for a particular ability (eg, mathematics, memorization, computer programming). These patients are referred to as Asperger, or autistic, savants.

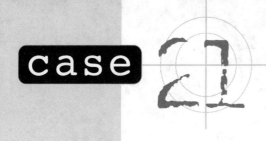

case 21

CC   A 6-year-old girl is brought to the pediatrician because she **refuses to go to school.**

HPI   As her mother drives her to school, she becomes very **distressed and cries, "Mommy, please don't leave me!"** She clings to her mother's legs and sobs hysterically. When asked what she is so worried about, she replies that she thinks her mother will get into a **car accident** or will be **kidnapped** and taken from the home. Her mother notes that her daughter **frequently complains of headaches or stomachaches on school days.**

case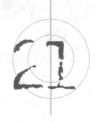

Separation Anxiety Disorder

Differential

GAD involves worry about many different things, not limited to a fear that something bad could happen to a major attachment figure.

Panic disorder is characterized by physical symptoms, including tachycardia, dyspnea, and dizziness. The trigger for a panic attack is usually not as clear as the imminent separation from an attachment figure that is seen in separation anxiety disorder.

Pervasive developmental disorders often include symptoms of anxiety, but they also feature prominent impairment of social skills not seen in children with separation anxiety disorder.

Pathogenesis

Separation anxiety disorder presents as overwhelming anxiety associated with separation from figures of attachment (usually parents), and often features **difficulty sleeping, nightmares,** and **physical complaints**. Patients typically present with **refusal to go to school** or **refusal to sleep alone at night**. Theories regarding the etiology of childhood separation anxiety disorder include the effects of genetics, temperament, and family dynamics.

Management

Typically, **CBT** and parental guidance are the basis of treatment for separation anxiety disorder. This approach includes firm but gentle limit-setting, elimination of secondary gain from staying home from school (watching TV, not doing schoolwork), relaxation training, evaluation of cognitive distortions ("My mom is going to be kidnapped while I'm at school"), gradual exposure to longer periods of time at school, and rewards for school attendance. Parents may have their own issues about separation or loss, and these should be thoughtfully explored. If the parent's issues are creating difficulty in separating from the child, the parent should be referred for individual treatment. If therapy does not result in a return to school, or if other mood or anxiety disorders are present, pharmacotherapy (typically an SSRI) could be indicated.

Breakout Point

> Separation anxiety is normal in children 8 months to 30 months of age.

case 22

CC A 14-year-old boy is brought to his pediatrician's office, but he **refuses** to leave the waiting room while his mother complains that "all he does is **argue and lose his temper.**"

HPI His mother goes on to lament that he seems to **purposefully disobey the rules** of the house and frequently refuses to do simple household chores, especially when he is asked. He **blames** his younger brother for his own mistakes and **becomes easily annoyed** by anyone in the family who talks to him. She feels frustrated, exhausted, and angry by his behavior. A recent report from his teacher noted that he is very **oppositional at school** as well; **frequently disrupting class, blatantly disobeying rules,** and **displaying an angry, spiteful attitude.**

case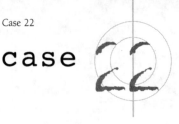

Oppositional Defiant Disorder (ODD)

Differential

Conduct disorder presents with serious behavior patterns in which the rights of others are violated. A diagnosis of conduct disorder precludes a diagnosis of ODD.

Major depressive disorder in children often presents with periods of irritability and noncompliance with rules; however, these periods are discrete and occur in the context of major mood symptoms.

ADHD may include noncompliance that results from inattention, impulsivity, and hyperactivity rather than a willful attitude.

Pathogenesis

ODD may be diagnosed in children who frequently lose their temper; argue with adults; refuse to comply with rules; **deliberately annoy people**; blame others for their mistakes; and are **often touchy, resentful, angry, or vindictive.** Symptoms must occur for a period of at least 6 months in a patient younger than 18 years of age. Maladaptive parenting techniques and poor parental relationships, either with the other parent or with the child, can lead to ODD.

Management

Multimodal treatment programs that include behavioral therapy, social skills training, conflict resolution, and problem-solving are most effective. Comorbid conditions (ADHD, mood disorders) may respond to pharmacotherapy and enhance compliance.

Breakout Point

> ODD is slightly more common in boys until 13 years of age, after which the diagnosis is equally common in boys and girls.

case 23

CC A 55-year-old **man** is brought to his primary care physician by his daughter following repeated episodes of falling.

HPI The daughter reports that her father constantly reeks of alcohol. The patient is **annoyed** by criticism of his drinking and feels that he drinks only on a social basis. He reports previous unsuccessful attempts to **cut down on his drinking** to prove that "it wasn't a problem." At times he admits to **feeling guilty** about his drinking but feels that there is nothing wrong with "a little **eye-opener** in the morning" or "a nightcap now and then." The daughter reports that her paternal uncles both passed away from alcoholic cirrhosis.

PE Significant for hepatomegaly, periumbilical varicosities, and hemorrhoids.

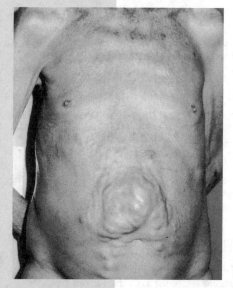

Figure 23-1. Periumbilical varicosities (caput medusae).

Labs LFTs: **AST and ALT elevated** with a ratio of >2:1.

Imaging CT, abdomen: hepatomegaly with fatty infiltration.

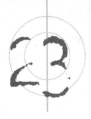

case 23

Alcohol Dependence

Differential

Alcohol dependence is diagnosed in patients who have had at least **three** of the following symptoms within the past year: **tolerance, withdrawal,** taking of the substance over a longer period of time or in greater amounts than intended, unsuccessful efforts to decrease use, spending a disproportionate amount of time obtaining the substance, reduction of important social or occupational activity, and use of alcohol in spite of persistent negative physical/psychological consequences. **Alcohol abuse** requires at least **one** of the following within the past year: impairment of major social or occupational role obligations, repeated use in hazardous situations, legal problems resulting from recurrent use, and continued use despite persistent negative interpersonal consequences.

Pathogenesis

Alcohol dependence results from changes in neurotransmitters and their receptors (most notably a downregulation of GABA receptors) due to chronic alcohol consumption. Subsequent abstinence from alcohol can result in tremors, confusion, seizures, and even death due to neuroexcitation. Genetic predisposition may impact the development of alcohol dependence.

Epidemiology

Males are affected two to three times more often than females.

Management

Individual and **group psychotherapy** as well as **peer-supervised 12-step groups** (ie, Alcoholics Anonymous) are vital to sustained sobriety. Various pharmacologic agents can also be helpful; disulfiram (Antabuse) inhibits the enzyme aldehyde dehydrogenase, Naltrexone is an opiate receptor antagonist. and acamprosate (Campral) are thought to act on the GABA and glutamate systems.

Complications

Medical complications affect almost every organ system and include **alcoholic cirrhosis** (with associated sequelae of **portal hypertension** including **caput medusae, esophageal varices, hemorrhoids,** and **spider angiomas**), pancreatitis, Wernicke-Korsakoff syndrome, alcoholic cardiomyopathy, aspiration pneumonia, iron and folate deficiency, gastritis, gastric ulcer, cerebellar degeneration, peripheral neuropathies, and a life-threatening withdrawal syndrome that involves seizures and DTs.

Breakout Point

> The **CAGE** questionnaire has been validated as a sensitive and specific tool for detecting problem drinking. Two or more positive answers indicate a likely diagnosis of alcohol dependence.
>
> Have you ever felt you should **C**ut down on your drinking?
> Have people **A**nnoyed you by criticizing your drinking?
> Have you ever felt bad or **G**uilty about your drinking?
> Have you ever had a drink first thing in the morning to steady your nerves or get rid of a hangover (**E**ye-opener)?

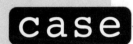
case
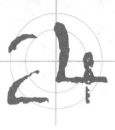

CC   A 21-year-old male college student comes to the ER with a complaint of "freaking out" after eating a brownie at a fraternity party.

HPI   He denies any loss of consciousness and is alert. He reports having felt "unreal," as though he were watching himself from the outside. He denies any hallucinations but does report feeling **paranoid** that someone might have been "tailing him." He reports that the 10-minute ride to the hospital "lasted 5 hours" and adds that he is **incredibly hungry.**

PE   VS: **tachycardia** (HR 105). PE: **dry mouth; injected conjunctiva.**

Labs   UA: **positive for THC** (will test positive for 7 to 10 days after use or up to 4 weeks in cases of heavy use).

case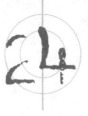

Cannabis Intoxication

Differential

Cocaine intoxication and **amphetamine intoxication** may present with anxiety, paranoia, and tachycardia but are typically associated with decreased appetite. Injected conjunctiva would be an unusual finding with cocaine or amphetamine intoxication.

Hallucinogen intoxication may present with anxiety, tachycardia, and diminished motor skills but most prominently involves vivid auditory, visual, and tactile hallucinations.

Pathogenesis

Delta-9-tetrahydrocannabinol (THC) is the active ingredient in marijuana and acts via the cannabinoid receptor. THC is highly lipophilic, which accounts for the fact that it may be detected up to 4 weeks after ingestion. Marijuana is most commonly smoked but can be ingested in brownies or "space cake." Intoxication is marked by diminished motor skills, impaired judgment, dry mouth, injected conjunctiva, paranoia, **distorted sense of time,** and increased appetite ("the munchies"). Chronic use may be associated with decreased fertility and **gynecomastia.** The existence of an amotivational syndrome due to chronic marijuana use is controversial.

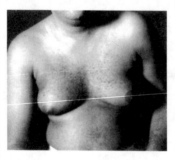

Figure 24-1. Gynecomastia.

Management

Education and **psychotherapy** to explore reasons for use. Individual and group psychotherapy may be useful in discussing abstinence issues and relapse prevention. In extreme cases, abstinence can be monitored by urine toxicology.

Breakout Point

Common Terms for Cannabis:	
Pot	Ganja
Weed	Chronic
Grass	Mary Jane
Reefer	

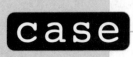
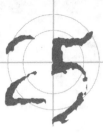

CC A **32-year-old man** is brought to the ER complaining of **severe chest pain.**

HPI On interview, the patient admits that he has been on a **cocaine binge.** About 1 month ago he **lost his job** after testing positive for cocaine on a urine toxicology screen; in addition, he was recently arrested on charges of cocaine possession. He claims to use cocaine only on weekends and has a history of fairly long periods of abstinence. He denies requiring escalating doses of the drug to reach his "high."

PE VS: hypertension (BP 168/110); tachycardia (HR 120). PE: dilated pupils, **perforated nasal septum.**

Labs Lytes/CBC: normal. Troponin I not elevated. ECG: sinus tachycardia with ST depression (evidence of ischemia). **Urine toxicology positive for cocaine** (will remain positive for 1 to 3 days).

case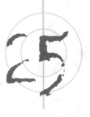

Cocaine Abuse

Differential

Cocaine dependence can be differentiated from cocaine abuse by the degree of social and work impairment, the presence of tolerance, or the occurrence of a withdrawal syndrome when the substance is stopped.

Pathogenesis

The acute behavioral effects of cocaine are related to **dopamine reuptake inhibition,** resulting in increased levels of dopamine and reinforcing reward-seeking behavior. Cocaine has potent mood-elevating effects, often resulting in **grandiosity** and a sense of **invulnerability.** Peripheral cardiovascular effects of cocaine are due to its sympathomimetic action.

Cocaine hydrochloride is usually formulated as a powder that can be snorted intranasally. Crystals of cocaine **freebase** (extracted from cocaine hydrochloride by processing with ammonia and ether) can be heated and the vapors inhaled. Cocaine hydrochloride can also be "cooked" with sodium bicarbonate to form **crack** cocaine, which is smoked from a glass pipe. Crack provides a more rapid and shorter-lived euphoria but is significantly cheaper. After cocaine binges, patients suffer "cocaine crash" (thought to be due to depletion of dopamine) and experience marked fatigue and increased appetite.

Management

Individual or group psychotherapy and peer-supervised 12-step programs form the foundation of treatment. **Pharmacotherapy remains experimental,** and there is currently no FDA-approved treatment; agents that have been used include amantadine, naltrexone, and anticonvulsants.

Complications

Life-threatening complications include cardiac **arrhythmias, myocardial infarction, cerebrovascular hemorrhage,** malignant hypertension, and seizure activity. Problems associated with chronic cocaine abuse include cocaine **cardiomyopathy** and necrosis of the nasal septum (due to vasoconstriction).

Breakout Point

Common Terms for Cocaine:
Coke
Snow
Blow
Candy
Speedball (a combination of cocaine and heroin)

case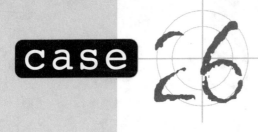

CC A 52-year-old man admitted 3 days ago for pneumonia complains of **tremor, insomnia,** and seeing "spiders crawling all over the walls."

HPI The patient is unable to give a coherent history; however, his medical record indicates a history of heavy drinking, and admission serum toxicology was positive for alcohol. He had earlier complained of **nausea** and had appeared **anxious** and **diaphoretic.** Tonight he seemed increasingly **confused,** becoming **paranoid** and **agitated,** accusing his nurse of trying to poison him.

PE VS: **tachycardia** (HR 120); **hypertension** (BP 210/100); tachypnea (RR 26); afebrile. PE: dilated pupils; **hyperreflexia; grossly tremulous.** On mental status exam, patient is **disoriented** to time and place; thought processes are grossly confused; patient appears to be responding to **visual hallucinations.**

Labs Lytes: normal. BUN and creatinine: normal. CBC: **macrocytic anemia.** LFTs: **elevated AST and ALT in 2:1 ratio.**

case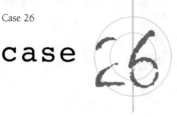

Alcohol Withdrawal

Differential

Substance-induced psychotic disorder may be differentiated from DTs by the absence of tremor, diaphoresis, and autonomic instability. Toxicology screening can also be helpful with the diagnosis.

Acute substance intoxication such as PCP and amphetamine intoxication can present with symptoms of autonomic hyperexcitability and confusion similar to DTs, although usually without tremor or diaphoresis. Toxicology screening can be important in distinguishing between the two.

Sedative/hypnotic withdrawal syndrome is nearly impossible to distinguish from acute alcohol withdrawal because the pathophysiologic mechanism is essentially the same; differentiation can be made via substance abuse history and urine toxicology.

Delirium due to a general medical condition can be distinguished via a thorough history and physical exam to identify underlying medical illnesses (eg, infections, metabolic abnormalities, stroke, tumor) that cause delirium.

Pathogenesis

Alcohol is thought to exert its psychotropic effects by hyperpolarizing neurons via agonism of the GABA receptor, producing GABA receptor down regulation with chronic consumption. Abrupt discontinuation of alcohol results in neuronal hyperexcitability that presents as **agitation, confusion, tremulousness, hallucinations, diaphoresis,** and **autonomic instability**—collectively known as alcohol withdrawal delirium or DTs.

Epidemiology

5% of all hospitalized alcoholic patients develop DTs.

Complications

The **mortality rate** from DTs has been estimated to be as **high** as 20% if left untreated, because it progresses to **seizures,** coma, and death. Mortality may also ensue from heart failure, infection, or injury sustained during seizure. Delirium typically occurs 2 to 7 days after the last drink, although other symptoms may present sooner.

Management

The mainstay of treatment is **benzodiazepine** administration and taper. Lorazepam (Ativan) may be useful in hepatic failure, because its metabolites are readily excreted without extensive liver metabolism. Patients should be well hydrated and given **parenteral thiamine** for 3 to 4 days. **Neuroleptics** may be used to manage severe agitation or psychosis.

Breakout Point

> The Clinical Institute Withdrawal Assessment for Alcohol (**CIWA-Ar**) scale is a validated tool used to rate the severity of symptomatic alcohol withdrawal and is often used as a measure in symptom triggered treatment of withdrawal.

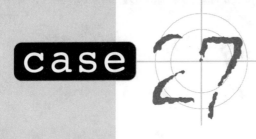

CC A **19-year-old** man is brought to the hospital by ambulance after jumping from the second floor window of his fraternity house.

HPI Fraternity brothers report that the patient appeared to be in a **dream-like state,** claiming to "hear colors" **(synesthesia),** and see kaleidoscopic patterns scroll across the walls. He appeared **restless** and told everyone that he was going to "fly to the ends of the world." On interview, the patient appeared **paranoid** and told the physician that people were trying to kill him.

PE VS: hypertension (BP 170/90); tachycardia (HR 110); tachypnea (RR 32); febrile. PE: diaphoretic and tremulous with mild abrasions throughout extremities; upper and lower extremity **hyperreflexia, lack of coordination, blurred vision,** and **dilated pupils.**

Labs Lytes/CBC: normal. BUN and creatinine: normal. UA: toxicology negative.

Imaging CT, spine: negative.

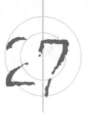

Lysergic Acid Diethylamide Intoxication

Differential

Substances such as **cocaine, amphetamine, and PCP** as well as **alcohol withdrawal** (DTs) can mimic some of the symptoms of LSD intoxication. A thorough history, urine toxicology, and physical exam can help identify the specific substance.

Psychotic illnesses such as **bipolar disorder, schizophrenia, and severe depression** are often difficult to distinguish from substance-induced psychosis, although substance related psychosis is more likely to present with visual and tactile (rather than auditory) hallucinations.

Pathogenesis

LSD or "acid" is a potent **serotonin agonist** with other poorly understood mechanisms of action, which has powerful hallucinogenic and psychedelic properties that peak at 2 to 3 hours and last up to 12 hours.

Prolonged psychotic symptoms can sometimes be seen in LSD abuse. Some individuals experience **"flashbacks"** during periods of abstinence, even years after their last use of LSD. Symptoms often include geometric hallucinations and other visual hallucinatory phenomena. "Bad trips" are marked by reactions to distressing psychotic symptoms.

Management

The primary treatment approach involves **decreasing sensory input** and keeping the patient safe until drug effects wear off. Assure the patient in a calm manner that he or she is safe and that his or her symptoms are a consequence of LSD (**"talking patient down"**). If agitation is severe, treatment with **neuroleptics** (haloperidol) or **benzodiazepines** (lorazepam, diazepam) may help.

Breakout Point

> LSD is typically formulated as a liquid that is then absorbed onto paper ("blotter") or gelatin ("windowpane") and taken by placing on the tongue.

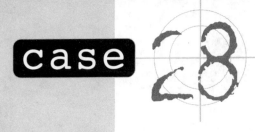

case 28

CC A 28-year-old man admitted 24 hours ago after being involved in a motor vehicle accident is complaining of **severe nausea** and **diarrhea.**

HPI The patient also reports **muscle aches, abdominal cramping,** and **anxiety.** Nursing staff note that he appears quite restless and is demanding to leave the hospital.

PE VS: **fever** (39.6°C); **hypertension** (BP 160/100); **tachycardia** (HR 104); tachypnea (RR 22). PE: significant **diaphoresis, rhinorrhea,** and **lacrimation.** Markedly **dilated pupils.** Diffuse **"gooseflesh"** (piloerection); multiple punctate lesions with thrombosed veins (**track marks**) over the antecubital fossae.

Labs Toxicology screen is positive for opiates.

case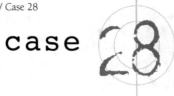

Opiate Withdrawal

Differential

Alcohol withdrawal is usually accompanied by significant confusion and lacks the hallmark symptoms of rhinorrhea, lacrimation, and piloerection seen in opiate withdrawal.

Infectious GI illnesses may present with a syndrome similar to opiate withdrawal. Careful history and physical examination, along with toxicology testing, are vital to accurate diagnosis.

Pathogenesis

Opiate receptors are broadly distributed throughout the CNS, peripheral nervous system, and GI tract; thus opiate withdrawal presents with prominent symptoms in each of these domains. Acute withdrawal symptoms begin approximately 8 hours after the last use, peak in 2 to 3 days, and may last up to 10 days. Some symptoms, such as insomnia and craving, can persist for up to 6 months following discontinuation.

Abused opiates include those available by prescription as well as the illicit drug heroin. Heroin can be snorted intranasally or injected intravenously ("shooting") or subcutaneously ("skin popping").

Management

Treatment should focus on opiate replacement and symptomatic management. **Methadone** is a long-acting opiate agonist that can be used for short-term detoxification or long-term maintenance treatment. **Buprenorphine** is a **partial agonist** at the opiate receptor that is approved for outpatient opiate detoxification. Levo-alpha acetylmethadol (LAAM) is a rarely used synthetic opiate with a half-life even longer than that of methadone.

Clonidine, an α_2-adrenergic agonist, suppresses the autonomic hyperactivity often seen in opiate withdrawal. Muscle cramps, abdominal cramps, diarrhea, and nausea should all be treated symptomatically. **Comorbid depression and anxiety** frequently occur and should also be addressed. In patients engaged in intravenous drug abuse, a thorough workup of infectious disease should be initiated with a focus on **HIV, hepatitis C,** and **bacterial endocarditis.**

Breakout Point

> **Prochaska and DiClemente's transtheoretical model of the stages of change** is often employed in addressing addictive behaviors. It has five stages:
> 1. **Precontemplation:** has no intention of taking action
> 2. **Contemplation:** intends to take action
> 3. **Preparation:** has taken some steps toward initiating change
> 4. **Action:** has acted to change behavior significantly
> 5. **Maintenance:** is working on maintaining changes that have been made

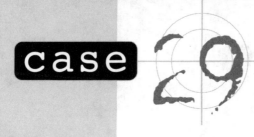

case

CC   A **25-year-old man** is brought to the ER by police after being arrested for **violently assaulting** a police officer.

HPI   Neighbors called police when they observed him **acting bizarrely**, shouting obscenities in the street while wearing only his boxer shorts. When police arrived, the patient became acutely **agitated and belligerent**, yelling "I'll take you all down!" Police report that the patient seemed "**immune to pain**," requiring five officers to restrain him.

PE   VS: hypertension (BP 170/100); tachypnea (RR 32); tachycardia (HR 126); fever (38.6°C). PE: neurologic exam reveals horizontal and **vertical nystagmus, ataxia,** dysarthria, **numbness** in upper and lower extremities, hyperreflexia, and **muscular rigidity;** mental status exam reveals gross **impairments in concentration, memory, and orientation.**

Labs   Lytes/CBC: normal. **Elevated serum CPK** (2000). UA: **myoglobinuria; urine toxicology positive for PCP.**

case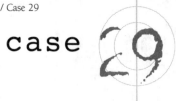

Phencyclidine Intoxication

Differential

Substances such as cocaine, amphetamine, and alcohol can mimic PCP psychosis. A thorough history, urine toxicology, and physical exam searching for signs of illicit drug use (nasal septum perforation, track marks) help identify the specific substance.

Psychotic illnesses such as bipolar disorder, schizophrenia, and severe depression are often indistinguishable from substance-induced psychosis. Although substance abuse may occur together with major psychiatric illnesses, careful longitudinal history, urine toxicology, and physical exam are key factors in their differentiation.

Pathogenesis

Symptoms of PCP intoxication are thought to result from interactions with multiple neurotransmitters, including antagonism at the PCP receptor of the ion-channel-gated **NMDA receptor complex**. Potentially fatal complications include hypertensive crisis, respiratory arrest, malignant hyperthermia, status epilepticus, and ARF secondary to **rhabdomyolysis** and **myoglobinuria**.

Management

Activated charcoal and **gastric lavage** may be indicated if the drug was taken orally (it can also be smoked). Acidification of the urine can accelerate clearance of the drug. Agitation can be controlled by **benzodiazepines** (lorazepam, clonazepam, diazepam), whereas more severe presentations with psychotic symptoms can be managed with **neuroleptics**. Mechanical restraints should be avoided as much as possible because of the increased risk of rhabdomyolysis, but this should be carefully weighed against the risk of injury to the patient or others stemming from agitation.

Breakout Point

> PCP was produced as a veterinary anesthetic. It is commonly referred to as "angel dust" and is a frequent adulterant of marijuana.

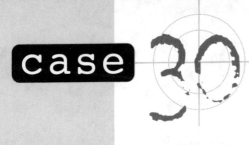

case

CC A 23-year-old woman is brought to the ER by ambulance after being found **unresponsive** by her roommate.

HPI The patient was found slumped on her bedroom floor, **breathing shallowly**, and not responding to her roommate's pleas for her to "wake up." Her roommate tearfully notes that the patient's new boyfriend is "a bad influence . . . he's on all sorts of drugs."

PE VS: **bradycardia** (to 52); **hypotension** (to 70/40); respirations shallow (rate of 6). Physical exam reveals an unresponsive young woman with **pinpoint pupils, mild perioral cyanosis, and multiple punctuate wounds** along the dorsum of her left foot.

Labs Toxicology screen positive for **opiates.**

case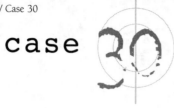

Opiate Intoxication

Differential

Medical causes of somnolence and confusion, including stroke, infection, seizure, and metabolic disturbance should be carefully investigated and ruled out.

Pathogenesis

Clinical hallmarks of opiate intoxication are profound sedation, slurred speech, pinpoint pupils (miosis), and respiratory depression (which can make the condition a medical emergency). Opiates are available in many different formulations including prescription medications (morphine, fentanyl, oxycodone, meperidine, hydromorphone, methadone) and the illegal drug heroin. Heroin may be snorted intranasally, smoked, or injected (either intravenously or subcutaneously). Patients may try to inject in unusual sites such as the feet, neck, or genitalia, either as a result of lost venous access elsewhere, or in an attempt to conceal their habit. Use of opiates, especially intravenously, is associated with a euphoric rush that prompts repeat use and addiction.

Management

Naloxone (Narcan) is an opioid antagonist that rapidly reverses opiate toxicity. In cases of overdose, **IV administration of naloxone immediately reverses sedation, respiratory depression, and unresponsiveness. Prolonged monitoring of the patient is indicated** because the short half-life of naloxone and longer action of many opiates can result in a re-emergence of respiratory suppression once the initial dose of naloxone is metabolized. In the opiate-dependent patient, naloxone precipitates withdrawal, frequently resulting in agitation (no matter what the cause of the patient's altered mental status, limiting the utility of naloxone as a diagnostic tool). Any comorbid psychiatric or medical illnesses should be addressed, with special attention to infectious diseases such as hepatitis C and HIV. Opportunities for ongoing addiction treatment should be offered to the patient.

Breakout Point

> Naloxone is often confused with naltrexone, an opioid antagonist available in oral formulation that is used in the long-term treatment of alcohol and drug addiction. Remember:
>
> Nal**OX**one treats hyp**OX**ia

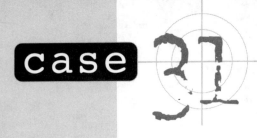

case

CC A 25-year-old man is brought to the ER by police after they were called in response to the sound of gunshots coming from his apartment.

HPI The patient appears **confused** and **agitated, speaking rapidly.** He seems to describe concern that "government agents" are trying to harm him. He notes hearing them in the crawl space above his apartment, prompting him to shoot into the ceiling.

PE VS: **tachycardia** (to 110); **hypertension** (to 160/95). Physical exam reveals an agitated young man, **rapidly pacing** around the examination room, gesticulating wildly with his hands. His **speech is rapid and pressured.** His thoughts are similarly rapid and tangential. On exam, his **teeth are in markedly poor condition,** with black and brown staining, and erosion and chipping of the enamel.

Labs Toxicology screen **positive for amphetamine.**

Imaging Not relevant.

case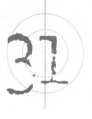

Amphetamine Intoxication

Differential

Cocaine intoxication can appear similar to amphetamine intoxication but does not usually feature the pronounced dental effects associated with methamphetamine. Careful history and exam along with toxicology screening is vital to diagnosis.

Schizophrenia or **bipolar disorder** may present with symptoms similar to amphetamine intoxication. Again, careful history and exam along with toxicology screening is vital to diagnosis.

Pathogenesis

Amphetamines have a stimulating effect and thus are frequently abused by those with a need to stay awake and alert (eg, long-distance truck drivers, students). Chronic amphetamine abuse can result in a syndrome that features symptoms of both psychosis and mania. Prominent **paranoia, agitation,** and **visual hallucinations** are features of amphetamine-induced psychosis. Amphetamines are available in a variety of formulations, including prescribed medications such as dextroamphetamine (Dexedrine) and methylphenidate (Ritalin). These are typically abused by grinding the tablets and snorting of the fragments intranasally. Methamphetamine abuse is a rapidly growing problem in the United States. The drug can be manufactured from readily available household chemicals without need for import or growth of a base ingredient. Methamphetamine can be snorted, smoked, or injected. **Bruxism** (teeth-grinding) is a frequent side effect of amphetamine use, often causing methamphetamine addicts to break or crack their teeth. Dental erosion is further exacerbated by the acidity of methamphetamine fumes which degrades dental enamel.

Management

Neuroleptics can be used in the initial stages of treatment to manage symptoms of psychosis. Benzodiazepines may also be used to minimize anxiety and agitation. Individual and group psychotherapy, along with peer-supervised 12-step groups, is vital to maintaining long-term abstinence.

Breakout Point

> The dental erosion associated with methamphetamine abuse is widely referred to as "meth-mouth."

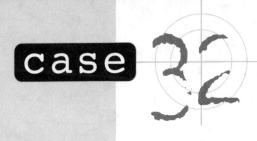

case 32

CC A 34-year-old woman presents to the ER complaining of **nausea,** diarrhea, **vomiting,** and **unsteady gait.**

HPI The patient has **a history of bipolar disorder** and has been treated with medication for the past 10 years. Yesterday she began feeling ill. She notes **blurred vision** and hand **tremor,** adding that she feels more **fatigued** than usual. This morning she felt dizzy and actually fell to the ground.

PE VS: tachycardia (HR 108); normal RR; **orthostatic hypotension** (BP 135/80 sitting and 110/70 standing); afebrile. PE: **dysarthria;** coarse hand tremors; **hyperreflexia** of upper and lower extremities; muscle **fasciculations;** impaired finger-to-nose coordination; **ataxic gait.**

Labs Lytes/CBC: leukocytosis. Lithium level of 2.9 (therapeutic levels 0.8 to 1.2). ECG: sinus tachycardia with T-wave inversion; regular rhythm with no evidence of ischemic changes.

case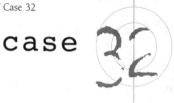

Lithium Toxicity

Differential

Delirium due to other substances must be part of differential diagnosis; careful physical exam and a toxicology screen are vital to timely diagnosis.

Pathogenesis

Lithium has been used as a medication since the 19th century, specifically for the treatment of mania since the mid-20th century. Lithium toxicity can result from overdose, dehydration, renal failure, or fluid shifts during pregnancy. Multiple medication interactions, notably thiazide diuretics, NSAIDS, and ACE inhibitors, can also elevate lithium levels.

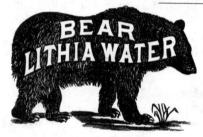

Figure 32-1. A historical advertisement for a lithium-containing medication.

Complications

Seizure, coma, nephrogenic diabetes insipidus, rash, acne, psoriasis, cardiac arrhythmias, weight gain, and hypothyroidism may result from lithium intoxication; permanent complications of intoxication include cerebellar ataxia and anterograde amnesia.

Management

Lithium should be held until levels return to within normal limits. If symptoms of intoxication are mild and the lithium level is less than 2.5, **IV fluid hydration** with normal saline should be started and electrolyte abnormalities corrected as long as there is no evidence of CHF or renal failure. Levels above 2.5, regardless of clinical symptoms, constitute a medical emergency. **Hemodialysis** should be used to rapidly decrease toxic lithium levels; even after dialysis, levels should be closely monitored because of re-equilibration from tissues. Factors that may have caused the acute increase in lithium level should be carefully evaluated.

Breakout Point

Potential Side Effects of Lithium (NAVAL WITCH)		
Nephrogenic Diabetes Insipidus	**L**eukocytosis	**C**ardiac Arrhythmia
Ataxia	**W**eight Gain	**H**ypothyroidism
Visual Changes	**I**tch (psoriasis)	
Acne	**T**remor	

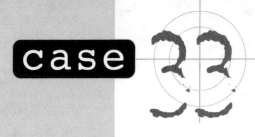

case 33

CC A 55-year-old white woman with treatment-refractory depression presents to the ER complaining of **throbbing headache, diaphoresis, anxiety, nausea, vomiting,** and **confusion.**

HPI She reports that over the past few years she has had trials of numerous antidepressants without benefit and was recently started on **phenelzine.** Last night, she went out to a cocktail party with friends, drank a glass of Chianti **wine,** and ate a few servings of **aged cheese.**

PE VS: **hypertension** (BP 210/120); tachypnea (RR 28); **tachycardia** (HR 124); fever (39.4°C). PE: neurologic exam reveals dilated pupils; neurologic exam otherwise normal.

Labs ECG: sinus tachycardia. Lytes/CBC: normal. BUN and creatinine normal. UA: urine toxicology negative.

Imaging CT, head: normal.

case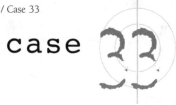

Hypertensive Crisis

Differential

Other causes of hypertension include uncontrolled primary hypertension, pheochromocytoma, thoracic aortic dissection, cocaine, amphetamines, neuroleptic malignant syndrome, and serotonin syndrome. A careful history and physical exam is essential in making the diagnosis.

Pathogenesis

Hypertensive crisis occurs with concomitant use of **MAO inhibitors (phenelzine** and **tranylcypromine)** and **tyramine-rich products** or **sympathomimetic medications** (eg, stimulants, decongestants). The metabolism of tyramine-containing foods is blocked by the inhibition of monoamine oxidase; the subsequent increase in circulating tyramine precipitates norepinephrine release, resulting in a **hyperadrenergic state.** Hypertensive crisis can result in potentially fatal complications including **stroke, myocardial infarction,** and **arrhythmias.**

Tyramine-rich foods include aged cheese products, fermented meats (sausage, salami), wine, beer, pickled herring, yogurt, beans, and yeast extracts. The concomitant use of MAO inhibitors and serotonergic agents (SSRIs, clomipramine) can result in serotonin syndrome; other potentially fatal interactions occur with **meperidine** and **dextromethorphan.**

All patients prescribed MAO inhibitors should receive extensive dietary education to prevent this potentially lethal reaction. Before starting an MAO inhibitor, a washout period from other antidepressants of at least five half-lives (usually about 2 weeks, but 5 weeks for fluoxetine) is recommended. Similarly, after stopping an MAO inhibitor, a **2-week washout period** should be observed before starting another antidepressant.

Management

Urgent pharmacologic management with either **IV phentolamine** (α-adrenergic antagonist) or **nifedipine** (calcium channel blocker) is vital. Beta-blockers should be avoided because they may result in unopposed α-mediated vasoconstriction, exacerbating hypertension. The MAO inhibitor should be held until the interacting agent has been cleared from the body.

Breakout Point

> **Selegiline** is a selective **MAO-B** inhibitor used in the treatment of Parkinson disease. At higher doses it also inhibits MAO-A, increasing the likelihood of interactions with foods and medication. The antibiotic **linezolid** also has some MAO-inhibiting properties.

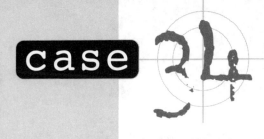

CC   A 37-year-old **woman** with chronic schizophrenia is noted by her psychiatrist to **involuntarily pucker her lips** and **grimace**.

HPI   Review of the medical record reveals the onset of **schizophrenia** 20 years ago and subsequent treatment with a variety of typical **neuroleptic medications**. She is currently prescribed haloperidol 10 mg twice daily and benztropine 1 mg twice daily, with excellent control of her hallucinations and paranoid delusions.

PE   Neurologic exam significant for **jerking movements** of her shoulders with **writhing** motion of the hands, **involuntary darting movements of the tongue**, and **lip smacking**.

Labs   Lytes/CBC: normal. TFTs: normal; RPR/VDRL nonreactive.

Imaging   CT, head: normal.

case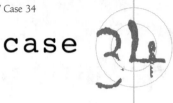

Tardive Dyskinesia (TD)

Differential

A variety of **movement disorders,** including Parkinson disease, Wilson disease, hemiballismus, or basal ganglia injury, may present with symptoms similar to TD. Careful history is vital to accurate diagnosis.

Pathogenesis

The precise cause of TD is unknown; however, neuroleptics have been postulated to **increase dopamine receptor sensitivity** in the striatum and produce neuron-damaging free radicals. TD does not always improve with discontinuation of neuroleptics.

The risk of TD **increases with the duration of neuroleptic use** (tardive means late-appearing). **Increasing age** is the greatest risk factor for TD. Other factors that may increase risk include female gender, the presence of a mood disorder, and organic brain disease.

Severe TD may result in marked **dysarthria,** dysphagia, and other debilitating neurologic abnormalities. Symptoms may cause **significant social debilitation.**

Management

After adequate risk/benefit assessment, a decision must be made to **continue the neuroleptic, discontinue the neuroleptic,** or to **switch to another neuroleptic.** If the decision is made to continue the current medication, **dose reduction** may be useful. When a decision is made to discontinue the neuroleptic, a slow taper is indicated, with careful monitoring for emergent psychotic symptoms. **During the early phase of the taper, TD may actually worsen before it begins to improve.** Switching to atypical neuroleptic agents such as olanzapine or risperidone may prove useful in the treatment of TD while continuing to control psychotic symptoms. Clozapine, which has the lowest association with TD, may also be used. Reduced risk of TD is one of the major benefits of the atypical neuroleptics.

Breakout Point

> All patients receiving chronic treatment with neuroleptics should undergo regular evaluation for involuntary movements. The **Abnormal Involuntary Movement Scale (AIMS)** is frequently used to assess and grade unusual movements.

case

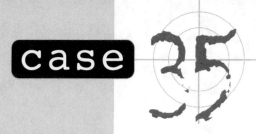

CC A psychiatrist receives a call from the hospital laboratory reporting that her patient, a **48-year-old woman** with chronic paranoid schizophrenia, has a **WBC of 3400.**

HPI This patient has been prescribed clozapine (Clozaril), an atypical neuroleptic, for 5 months. She gets a **weekly CBC with differential.** Until now, her WBC has been within the normal range. The psychiatrist asks the patient to come to her office that day to discuss this result.

PE VS: normal. Physical exam is normal.

Labs WBC 3400, differential: neutrophils 55%, band neutrophils 5%; absolute neutrophil count (ANC): 2040.

case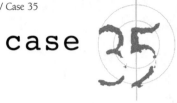

Agranulocytosis

Differential

Immunosuppression due to medical illness or the **effects of other medications** should be considered in the differential diagnosis of decreases in the WBC or ANC.

Pathogenesis

Monitoring for clozapine therapy includes a **WBC every week for the first 6 months of therapy and every other week thereafter** for the duration of treatment. Agranulocytosis is a serious side effect that has limited the use of this particularly effective neuroleptic. Patients treated with clozapine are followed by the Clozaril National Registry.

Management

The parameters for monitoring clozapine are as follows:

1. **If WBC decreases more than 3000 from the last test or decreases on three consecutive tests,** twice-weekly monitoring of CBC with differential is required but treatment may continue.
2. **If WBC is 3000 to 3500** (as with this patient), twice-weekly monitoring of CBC with differential is required but treatment may continue.
3. **If WBC is 2000 to 3000 or ANC is 1000 to 1500,** clozapine is stopped and CBC with differential is checked. Hospitalization may be necessary, but once the WBC normalizes, clozapine may be restarted.
4. **If WBC is less than 2000 or ANC is less than 1000,** clozapine is stopped, and the patient is hospitalized and placed in isolation. **Clozapine can never be restarted.**

Breakout Point

ANC = WBC × [percent neutrophils + percent band neutrophils]

case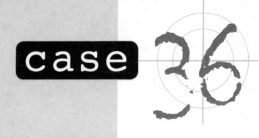

CC A 34-year-old man with a history of **schizophrenia** is brought to the hospital from his group home due to **agitation** and **disorientation.**

HPI Three days prior to presentation he had been discharged from an inpatient psychiatric unit on a **new high-potency neuroleptic medication.** Yesterday, his outpatient psychiatrist **increased the dose.** This morning, he was noted to be speaking loudly, stumbling, and appearing confused.

PE VS: fever (to 40°C), pulse 120, BP 155/80, and RR of 22. On exam he is profusely **diaphoretic** and unresponsive to verbal cues. Passive movement of his limbs reveals stable rigid resistance throughout the range of motion (**lead pipe rigidity**).

Labs Serum and urine toxicology: negative. UA: normal. CBC: **leukocytosis** to 13,000. LFTs: slightly elevated (ALT: 72; AST: 99). **CPK elevated** to 1346. Lytes reveal **metabolic acidosis.** LP: unremarkable.

Imaging CT, head: normal.

case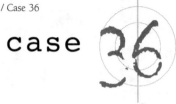

Neuroleptic Malignant Syndrome (NMS)

Differential

Serotonin syndrome may present with symptoms similar to NMS, though it usually features prominent myoclonus and typically lacks lead pipe rigidity.

Catatonia can feature rigidity and unusual posturing but does not generally present with fever, leukocytosis, or autonomic instability.

Malignant hyperthermia is closely related to NMS but occurs in the setting of volatile anesthetic exposure.

Pathogenesis

NMS, a complication of neuroleptic treatment, is a medical emergency. It can occur anytime during treatment, but is most often seen in the **first few weeks of treatment** and at **higher doses of high potency neuroleptics**. NMS is often seen in **younger patients** but can be seen in any age group at any point in the course of neuroleptic treatment.

The precise mechanism of NMS is unclear, but it is suspected that **decreased dopamine activity in the CNS** plays a significant role. It can present with a spectrum of symptoms including mental status changes, **muscle rigidity**, tremor, sustained muscle contractions (dystonia), paucity of movement (akinesia), mutism, diaphoresis, incontinence, dyskinesias, and dysphagia. **Autonomic instability** is also often prominent with **hyperthermia**, tachycardia, tachypnea, and labile BP. Laboratory findings typically show **elevated CPK, leukocytosis,** elevated LFTs, and various electrolyte abnormalities.

Complications

Prominent complications include **rhabdomyolysis,** seizure, hepatic failure, and DIC.

Management

Rapid recognition of NMS is essential, because mortality rates are estimated to be between 10% and 20%. **The offending medication should be immediately discontinued.** Treatment focuses on symptomatic measures such as hydration, **cooling, controlling hypertension,** and stabilizing respiratory and cardiac function. Treatment may also include administration of dopamine agonists **(bromocriptine, amantadine),** or the muscle relaxant **dantrolene.**

Breakout Point

Cardinal Symptoms of NMS (FEVER)
Fever
Encephalopathy
Vital Sign Instability
Elevation of WBC and CPK
Rigidity

case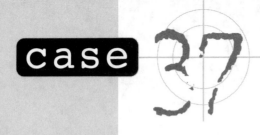

CC An 18-year-old female college student is brought to the ER after her roommates found her on the bathroom floor with an empty bottle of pills.

HPI Although she is **confused** on mental status exam, she is able to recall that she had a fight with her boyfriend at a party earlier and she had taken "all of the pills left" of a medication prescribed for "mild depression." She states that she had "cried herself to sleep" on the bathroom floor. She currently feels **"nauseated," "really warm,"** and **"restless."** She then tells the interviewer to "leave her alone." **She denies taking any other medications or substances.**

PE VS: fever (to 38.5°C), tachycardia (HR to 111), BP: 130/70. On exam, the patient is **markedly diaphoretic** and **shivering.** Neurological exam reveals **hyperreflexia, tremor, myoclonus, and dilated pupils (mydriasis).** Mental status exam reveals gross confusion and irritability.

Labs WBC elevated to 12,000. Lytes, LFTs, and urine toxicology are all normal.

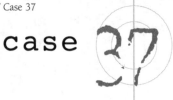

case

Serotonin Syndrome

Differential

Neuroleptic malignant syndrome (NMS) presents with the hyperthermia and confusion that may seen in serotonin syndrome, but NMS also features prominent rigidity, leukocytosis, and elevation of CPK. NMS is not typically associated with myoclonus.

Anticholinergic toxicity also presents with hyperthermia, mydriasis, and confusion but also usually features cutaneous flushing, dry skin and mucous membranes, functional ileus, and urinary retention. Careful history with special attention to medication history is vital to accurate diagnosis.

Pathogenesis

Serotonin syndrome is a condition caused **by excess serotonergic activity in the CNS**. It is **potentially life threatening** and is often caused by accidental or intentional **overdose of serotonergic medications**, or by **medication interactions** (especially SSRIs and MAO inhibitors).

Characteristics of serotonin syndrome include **mental status changes** (delirium, agitation/irritability, confusion, and restlessness), **neurological symptoms** (myoclonus, tremor, hyperreflexia, mydriasis, and hypertonia), and **autonomic symptoms** (hyperthermia, diaphoresis, tachycardia, and hypertension). Nausea, vomiting, and diarrhea may also occur. Laboratory findings are nonspecific.

Management

Serotonergic agents should be avoided, and a **complete medication list must be obtained.** Treatment occurs in an acute medical setting and is generally supportive, typically including hydration, vital sign monitoring, support of cardiovascular and respiratory status, and cooling if hyperthermia is present. **Benzodiazepines** may provide sedation. If the patient does not improve, **medications with serotonin antagonist properties** may be used (eg, cyproheptadine).

Breakout Point

Common Drugs and Drug Classes with Serotonergic Properties	
SSRIs	Sumatriptan
Monoamine Oxidase Inhibitors	Trazodone
Tricyclic Antidepressants	Dextromethorphan
Serotonin-Norepinephrine Reuptake Inhibitors (venlafaxine, duloxetine)	Amphetamines
	Cocaine
Lithium	Meperidine (Demerol)

case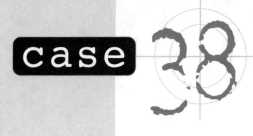

CC A 24-year-old man presents to a psychiatrist's office following hospitalization for his first manic episode. He states, "I don't know what to do, **I can't stop moving, I feel so restless. I can't stand it.**"

HPI During the interview he **stands up repeatedly, paces back and forth** in the office, and is too distracted to effectively participate in the exam. Prior to his hospitalization the patient had not been prescribed psychotropic medications. During his week on the inpatient unit, he was **started on risperidone** and lithium. His hospital discharge summary notes that after 5 days on the unit, his psychotic symptoms had resolved but **he still seemed agitated.** The **risperidone was increased** further, and it was thought that he was stable enough to be discharged.

PE On exam the patient is shifting in his chair, **swinging his legs** and looking down at the floor. The remainder of the physical exam is normal.

Labs CBC/Lytes: normal.

case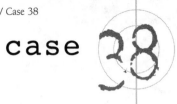

Akathisia

Differential

Symptoms of restlessness associated with various psychiatric illnesses such as agitated depression, psychosis, anxiety disorders, substance withdrawal/intoxication, dementia, or delirium may appear similar to akathisia.

Pathogenesis

Akathisia is a **subjective sense of restlessness** that can start within several weeks of starting or increasing a neuroleptic. Akathisia is **more common with typical neuroleptics** but also occurs with atypical neuroleptics. Akathisia may manifest with **agitation, pacing, fidgeting, trouble sitting,** or **difficulty standing still.**

Akathisia may be mistaken for agitation due to psychosis, resulting in an increase in neuroleptic dose, inadvertently exacerbating the symptoms.

Management

Beta-blockers (propranolol) are the primary treatment for akathisia. Benzodiazepines and clonidine can also be used.

Breakout Point

> Although anticholinergic medications are the treatment of choice for neuroleptic side effects such as parkinsonism and acute dystonia, they are less effective for treatment of akathisia.

case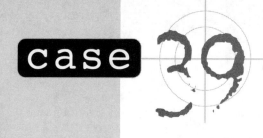

CC A **17-year-old boy** presents to the hospital requesting "an x-ray of the brain."

HPI The patient has concerns about a "machine in his head" controlled by the cellular phones of his teachers. When the emergency physician refuses to order the requested study, the patient becomes acutely agitated, requiring one dose of haloperidol 10 mg intramuscularly. Shortly after receiving the medication, he is found writhing in pain, clutching his neck, with his **head turned far to one side.**

PE VS normal. On exam, sustained muscle contraction of the neck is noted, although the rest of his body is not affected. Remainder of physical and neurologic exam is normal.

Labs Serum and urine toxicology negative.

case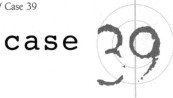

Acute Dystonia

Differential

Neurologic conditions such as **seizures, meningitis, tetanus,** and primary dystonias may present with similar body positioning. **Catatonia** may also present with abnormal posturing. A thorough medication history is vital to the diagnosis.

Pathogenesis

Acute dystonia is a sustained muscle contraction of variable duration that results in a **markedly abnormal positioning of a part of the body.** Affected body parts may include the **deviation of the neck to the back or side** (retrocollis, **torticollis**), **jaw spasm** (trismus), dysphagia, impaired speaking or breathing due to laryngeal spasm, **tongue protrusion,** abnormal twisting of the limbs or trunk, and **eye deviation in any direction** (oculogyric crisis). The mechanism of neuroleptic-induced acute dystonia is not well understood, but may involve the balance of the cholinergic and dopaminergic activity in the basal ganglia.

Incidence is particularly high in men and individuals younger than 30 years of age. Acute dystonia **occurs within days after treatment has commenced** or as the dose is being rapidly increased. It is most often seen with **high doses of high-potency neuroleptics** such as haloperidol, fluphenazine, thiothixene, and trifluoperazine.

Management

Treatment consists of administration of anticholinergic medication **(diphenhydramine, benztropine).** If there is no response, a benzodiazepine (lorazepam) may be given. The offending medication should be decreased or discontinued, possibly switching to an atypical neuroleptic, which is associated with lower incidence of dystonia. It is important to note that **laryngeal dystonia is a medical emergency** and requires ongoing monitoring and management of the airway.

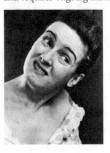

Figure 39-1. Torticollis.

Breakout Point

Anticholinergic agents are often coadministered with high-potency neuroleptics to provide prophylaxis against acute dystonia. A "5, 2, 1" is shorthand for haloperidol 5 mg, lorazepam 2 mg, and benztropine 1 mg, a combination frequently used intramuscularly as an emergency chemical restraint.

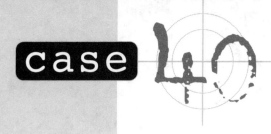

CC An agitated **72-year-old woman** is admitted to the ICU with **CHF** and pneumonia.

HPI She is started on a **quinolone antibiotic** for the pneumonia, **diuretics** for the CHF, and an **atypical neuroleptic** for the agitation. Hours later a code is called because of an arrhythmia detected on telemetry.

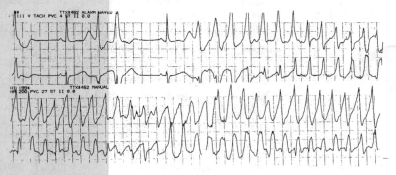

Figure 40-1. Patient's ECG.

PE Not relevant.

Labs Lytes: **hypokalemia** to 2.9 and **hypomagnesemia** to 1.2. CBC: moderate leukocytosis.

case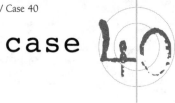

QTc Prolongation

Differential

Cardiac arrhythmias other than **torsades de pointes** (TDP) are distinguished by their morphology on ECG.

Pathogenesis

TDP is a form of polymorphic VT associated with **prolongation of the QTc interval**. Multiple medications are associated with QTc prolongation, including both typical neuroleptics (haloperidol, droperidol, thioridazine) and atypical neuroleptics (olanzapine, quietapine, risperidone). Medication induced QTc prolongation is thought to occur by **blockade of the flow of potassium ions** responsible for cardiac repolarization. Risk factors for QTc prolongation and TDP include **older age; female gender;** bradycardia; **LVH;** cardiac ischemia; and electrolyte abnormalities, including hypokalemia and hypomagnesemia.

Management

Development of TDP can be forestalled by **careful monitoring of QTc, potassium, and magnesium** for all patients receiving agents associated with QTc prolongation. If TDP does occur, appropriate advanced cardiac life support protocols should be followed to correct the arrhythmia. Once the patient is stabilized, the medication list should be thoroughly reviewed and QTc prolonging agents minimized or (if possible) discontinued.

Breakout Point

Other Agents That Are Associated with QTc Prolongation
Quinolone Antibiotics
Erythromycin
Methadone
Amiodarone
Quinidine

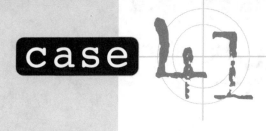

case 41

CC An **18-year-old female** college student presents to her gynecologist after **missing her last six periods**. She also reports being unable to tolerate the cold weather in Massachusetts and thinks she is **losing her hair**.

HPI Despite appearing cachectic, she feels **anxious about her weight** and **believes she is fat**. She significantly **restricts her diet** and **exercises for several hours a day**.

PE VS: **hypothermia** (35.6°C); **bradycardia** (HR 52); mild **hypotension** (BP 105/66); height 170 cm (67 in); weight 41.7 kg (92 lb; 68% of ideal body weight). PE: thin, emaciated young female; skin dry and scaly with downy body hair; slight pedal edema; neurologic exam normal.

EATING DISORDERS

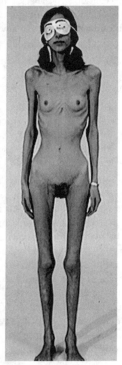

Figure 41-1. Emaciation.

Labs CBC: anemia; leukopenia. Lytes: hypokalemia. Hypoalbuminemia.

case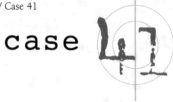

Anorexia Nervosa

Differential

Bulimia nervosa can be distinguished from anorexia based on criteria that an anorexic patient's body weight fall below the 85th percentile. Although binging and purging are central to bulimia nervosa, they may be features of anorexia and accordingly be diagnosed as anorexia nervosa, binge-eating/purging type.

Body dysmorphic disorder may have features of distorted body image but is distinguished from anorexia nervosa on the basis of body weight and prominent maladaptive eating/exercising behaviors.

Pathogenesis

The etiology of anorexia nervosa is thought to involve an interplay of biology, cultural factors, acute precipitating stressors, and maladaptive behavioral/psychological patterns. Cardinal features include intense **fear of weight gain, distorted body image, < 85% of ideal body weight,** and **amenorrhea.**

Epidemiology

Average **age at onset is between 14 and 18 years.** Anorexia nervosa is 10 to 20 times **more common in females** than males, and it is significantly more common in industrialized nations than in developing countries.

Complications

Complications include hypothermia, fluid/electrolyte abnormalities, edema (due to hypoalbuminemia), **osteoporosis,** endocrine abnormalities, anemia, leukopenia, hypotension, cardiac arrhythmias, and death (10% to 20% of hospitalized patients die within 10 to 30 years).

Management

Supportive measures for electrolyte disturbances, cardiovascular compromise, and renal insufficiency. **Hospitalization** is indicated in patients with significant metabolic derangements, cardiac arrhythmias, or body weight below the 75th percentile. **Cognitive behavioral interventions** are the mainstay of long-term treatment. Close supervision of caloric intake is important and is often reinforced with behavioral incentives. Patients who fail to gain weight may require bed rest and **tube feeding.** Caloric intake must be gradually increased to avoid **refeeding syndrome** (hypophosphatemia and hypomagnesemia due to increased cellular uptake) that can present with a variety of cardiac and neurologic symptoms and result in death. SSRIs may be used to treat comorbid symptoms of depression and anxiety.

Breakout Point

> Lanugo is fine, downy hair that appears on the bodies of patients with anorexia nervosa, likely in reaction to chronic hypothermia.

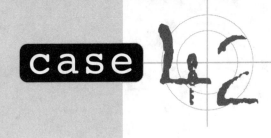

CC A **17-year-old girl** is brought to a psychiatrist by her parents for **worsening self-esteem** and **repeated attempts at "fad diets."**

HPI When interviewed alone, the girl confides that her troubles began when she started high school and became self-conscious about her weight. She now sneaks into the kitchen to **consume a tremendous amount of food** in a **short period of time.** She feels as though she **loses control of her eating** during these episodes. Afterward, she feels disgusted with herself and **induces vomiting** by sticking her fingers down her throat. At times she has "felt depressed" after vomiting but has not had any changes in sleep, energy, interest, or concentration. This behavior has persisted **at least twice a week for 3 months.**

PE **Eroded enamel** over front teeth; bilaterally **enlarged parotid glands** on palpation; extremities notable for multiple callus formation on backs of hands and knuckles.

Labs Lytes: hypokalemia; hypochloremia; elevated bicarbonate. CBC: normal. BUN, creatinine, vitamin B_{12}, folate, and TFTs: normal; RPR/VDRL nonreactive.

case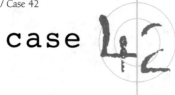

Bulimia Nervosa

Differential

Bulimia nervosa, nonpurging type meets the criteria of bulimia nervosa but without any purging behaviors (induced vomiting, laxative abuse, or enema use). The nonpurging type is typically associated with behaviors such as excessive exercise or fasting.

Anorexia nervosa can be distinguished from bulimia based on weight. In anorexia, the patient's weight must be < 85% of that expected for age and height.

Pathogenesis

The central feature of bulimia nervosa is repeated binge eating with subsequent inappropriate compensatory behavior (vomiting, excessive exercise, and misuse of diuretics, laxatives, or enemas). Psychological theories regarding the cause of the disorder include developmental arrest, familial conflict, and pressure to be thin secondary to societal factors. No definite biological etiology has been identified, although the norepinephrine and serotonin systems have been implicated.

Epidemiology

Average age of onset is 13 to 18 years; affects approximately 1% to 3% of women in industrialized countries. **Females** are affected more often than males.

Complications

Medical complications include dental caries, **hypokalemia, metabolic alkalosis,** esophagitis, Mallory-Weiss tear, **arrhythmias,** and death. Erosion of dental enamel occurs with repeated exposure to gastric acid with induced vomiting.

Management

Even in the absence of a major depressive episode, **antidepressants** are the mainstay of pharmacologic treatment. Bupropion (Wellbutrin) is contraindicated because of the increased risk of seizures in the setting of electrolyte imbalance. Various **psychotherapeutic modalities** (eg, **CBT** and family psychotherapy) have also been shown to be useful in the treatment of bulimia. **Hospitalization** is necessary in cases of severe electrolyte disturbance or other medical complications associated with bulimia.

Breakout Point

> **Russell sign** is the eponymous description of scarring and calluses found on the dorsum of the hand due to repeated exposure to gastric acid.

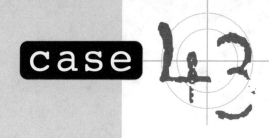

case 42

CC   A 72-year-old man with **progressive dementia** is admitted to the hospital after an episode of syncope. On workup, he is found to be markedly anemic, and his stool is guaiac-positive. He is refusing any further workup and asking to leave the hospital, despite extensive discussion of the likelihood of further morbidity and mortality.

HPI   On interview, the patient states, "I'll be fine, I need to go home to rake the yard." When asked why he was admitted to the hospital, he notes "I just got dizzy because of the heat." He goes on to state, "All of the doctors are talking about blood in my stool, but I haven't seen any. I think I just need to drink more water."

PE   He is alert and oriented to person, place, and time. He has some moderate deficits of short-term memory.

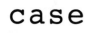 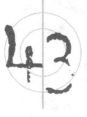

Capacity

Management

Capacity is a measure of a patient's ability to effectively make and express a consistent decision about their care based on an adequate understanding of the **facts of their condition** and of the "downstream" **consequences of their decision** in the setting of a discussion of **informed consent** with their physician. Capacity can (and should) be assessed by physicians of any specialty, but psychiatric consultation may be helpful in difficult cases, or in cases involving psychiatric illness. The assessment of capacity is specific to the decision being made; for instance a patient may have the capacity to make a reasonable decision regarding their dietary choices but would not be able to effectively understand the risks and benefits of a complex surgical procedure. In instances when a patient is deemed to lack capacity, the decision is referred to a previously designated **health care proxy** or **power of attorney** (if one exists). In the absence of such an advance directive, family and close associates are typically consulted. In some cases, it may be necessary to have the courts appoint a guardian for the patient. In difficult or controversial cases, discussion with the hospital legal counsel or a referral to the hospital ethics committee can also be useful.

Breakout Point

> **Competency** is a legal construct that describes a person's global ability to make decisions for himself or herself. A judgment of competency can only be made by the courts.

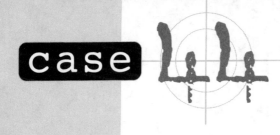

case

CC A 14-year-old girl is brought to her family physician by her mother for evaluation of amenorrhea for the past 2 months; she is subsequently found to have a positive pregnancy test.

HPI The patient asks the physician not to inform her mother of the results of the test. Later, the mother calls to ask if her daughter is pregnant.

PE Pelvic exam normal.

Labs Positive β-hCG.

case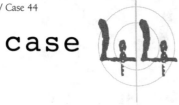

Disclosure of Teen Pregnancy

Management

The patient's confidentiality should be respected; however, disclosure to the parents by the minor should be encouraged. According to the AMA Code of Ethics, when a **minor (age < 18 years) seeks medical services, confidentiality should be maintained except when state law requires otherwise** (e.g., abortion in some states). It is, however, recommended that physicians explore the reasons for nondisclosure and facilitate problem solving. It is important to note that confidentiality should be broken to prevent serious harm to the minor or when parental involvement is necessary for treatment decisions. If sexual abuse is suspected, physicians are legally required to report to an appropriate protective agency (not to the parents). Sometimes such situations are ambiguous and require that the physician weigh and balance conflicting duties. Most hospitals have an ethics committee in which such quandaries can be discussed without revealing the identity of the patient. This resource can be helpful in making more informed and thoughtful choices in a difficult situation.

Breakout Point

> Classic cases in which confidentiality should be strictly maintained include **contraception, STDs, substance abuse, mental illness, and pregnancy.**

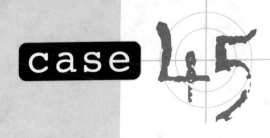
case 45

CC   A 32-year-old HIV-positive woman, now 24 weeks' pregnant, stopped taking AZT because it made her feel nauseous. Her physician is unsure whether this represents neglect.

HPI   Although the patient is informed that taking the medication can reduce the risk of HIV transmission to the fetus from 24% to 8%, she continues to refuse to take the medication.

case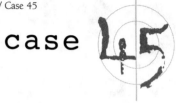

Fetal Neglect

Management

Cases involving withholding treatment that would affect a fetus (and not a newborn) do not constitute child abuse in the current U.S. legal system; hence, the wishes of the mother must be respected. A psychiatric consult might be indicated for an evaluation of capacity and to explore the mother's thinking. Her fear and confusion merit empathic support, and her decision may change in the context of an alliance that helps clarify her thinking.

Breakout Point

> Unlike refusal of medical treatment, use of illicit drugs while pregnant may be grounds for action by child welfare agencies.

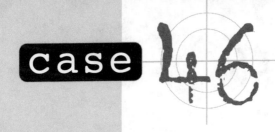

case 46

CC   A 24-year-old man with renal failure due to diabetic nephropathy has been doing well on dialysis for 6 months while awaiting an organ donor.

HPI   He now wishes to discontinue treatment despite his understanding that he will die without it. Although a psychiatric interview reveals no evidence of a mood or thought disorder, the patient's wife and mother request that dialysis be continued.

case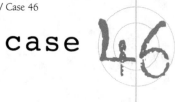

Withdrawal of Care

Management

In this case, because the patient is an **adult with capacity to decide which treatment to accept or deny,** his wishes should be respected. It is important to note that the **AMA Code of Ethics does not recognize an ethical distinction between withholding treatment** (never starting it) **and withdrawing treatment** (stopping midcourse). The law does, however, distinguish between withholding or withdrawing treatment (which is acceptable) and providing medications with the intent of helping a terminally ill patient hasten death (which is actionable). Finally, a physician who respects the patient's wish to die should attend to comfort care **(palliation)** and affirm the dying process. Psychiatric consultation can be helpful to rule out conditions that may be unduly influencing the patient's decision. The differential diagnosis may be quite broad and, above all else, should include delirium, particularly in hospitalized medical or surgical patients. The inherent altered level of consciousness in delirium often leads patients to make decisions without full appraisal of the consequences. Treatable conditions such as adjustment disorders and major depression should also be considered.

Breakout Point

> Use of high doses of opiates to ease respiratory distress in the dying patient is considered ethically justified even though it will hasten death, because death is not the intent of the treatment.

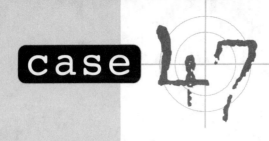

case **47**

CC   A 32-year-old female surgery resident is treated for a gunshot wound at the same hospital in which she is completing her residency.

HPI Later, the surgical chief resident asks the attending physician if he can look at her chart to ascertain when she will be ready to take calls again.

case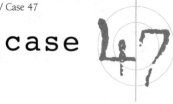

Patient–Doctor Confidentiality

Management

Confidential patient records should not be released without patient consent. Aspects of patient care should be discussed only with those who are directly involved in that case, not with friends, relatives, or colleagues. If confidentiality is breached, it is the duty of the physician to **inform** the patient.

Breakout Point

> The Health Insurance Portability and Accountability Act **(HIPAA)** is a federal law that sets out strict guidelines for the management and release of confidential health care information. Among other things, it requires the secure disposal of paper records and a signed waiver from the patient before any of their information can be disclosed. It can be permissible to disclose information without a waiver in emergency situations.

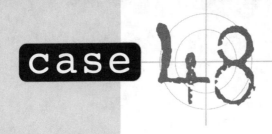

case **48**

CC A college student is referred for emergent psychiatric evaluation by his primary care physician after reporting that his political science instructor had rejected his romantic advances, stating "If I can't have her, no one will; I'm going to kill her."

HPI While awaiting transfer to the ER, the patient disappears and the physician is unable to locate him.

ETHICS

case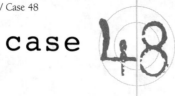

Tarasoff Decision

Management

Physicians are required by law to take appropriate steps to protect potential victims including **warning the potential victim, notifying the police** and/or **detaining the patient via commitment procedures.** This duty is described in the precedent-setting case of *Tarasoff v Regents of the University of California*, 551 P.2d 334 (1976). **There is no doctor–patient confidentiality standard that supersedes the duty to report imposed by the Tarasoff ruling.**

Breakout Point

> The Tarasoff case produced two rulings. *Tarasoff I* described a physician's duty to warn a potential victim. This was later superseded by *Tarasoff II*, which expanded the physician's duty to enacting measures to effectively **protect** a potential victim (which may still include a warning).

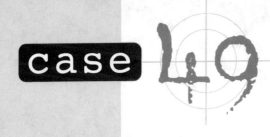
CC A neonate with Down syndrome is born with duodenal atresia.

HPI Although the parents are told that the atresia is surgically correctable and that the newborn will die without treatment, they request that treatment be withheld.

Imaging

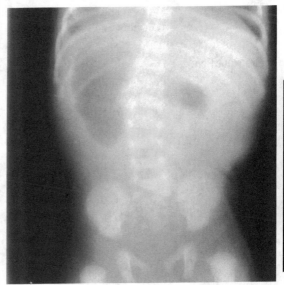

Figure 49-1. Abdominal film showing duodenal atresia with gas in the stomach and dilated duodenal bulb, but no gas in the distal GI tract.

ETHICS

97

case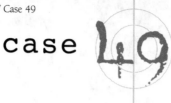

Withholding Treatment

Management

Do not withhold treatment. According to the AMA Code of Ethics, treatment **decisions must be made in the neonate's or child's best interests** rather than being based on the desires of the parents. Treatment can be withheld or withdrawn when there is little potential for success, when the risks outweigh the benefits, and when treatment will only extend the child's life such that suffering will exceed any possibilities for a meaningful existence. **Withholding of treatment is a form of neglect** that mandates reporting to social services (as for child abuse).

Breakout Point

> Down syndrome (trisomy 21) is the most common **genetic** cause of mental retardation. Fragile X syndrome is the most common **inherited** cause of mental retardation.

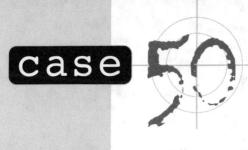

case 50

CC   A 26-year-old **woman** with a history of **unexplained hypoglycemia** presents with weakness and confusion.

HPI   She reports three previous episodes of hypoglycemia, **all occurring at other hospitals.** She is currently employed as a **nurse's aide** and lives with her sister, who has IDDM. Five years ago she had an exploratory laparotomy for abdominal pain, which revealed no explanation for her symptoms.

PE   VS: fever (38°C); tachycardia (HR 105); tachypnea (RR 22). PE: tremor; diaphoresis; diffuse abdominal tenderness.

Labs   Glucose low (25 mg/dL); elevated serum insulin (95 U/mL) with **decreased C-peptide** (<0.4 ng/mL) and **insulin antibodies present** (indicators of exogenous insulin).

case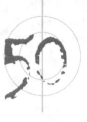

Factitious Disorder

Differential

Malingering also involves symptoms that are feigned, but the motivation is for secondary gain (eg, money, narcotics, housing, avoiding legal perils) other than assuming the sick role.

Somatoform disorders are characterized by multiple unexplained somatic symptoms that are not intentionally produced.

Pathogenesis

Factitious disorder is marked by the deliberate feigning or eliciting of symptoms of medical illness, with **assumption of the sick role** as the sole motivation. Cases have included administration of exogenous insulin to induce hypoglycemia, deliberate infection of surgical wounds with feces, and use of vanilla extract to mimic the laboratory findings of pheochromocytoma.

Epidemiology

Factitious disorder has been estimated to account for up to 6% of hospital admissions. **Health care workers** and **women** are disproportionately represented in this patient population.

Complications

Unnecessary medical evaluations and invasive procedures can account for significant morbidity and waste of health care funds. Careful documentation and effective coordination between health care providers may reduce these complications.

Management

Supportive, **nonaccusatory**, and **empathic confrontation** is often employed. Long-term psychotherapy may be used but success is limited. No pharmacotherapy has been proven useful.

Breakout Point

Factitious disorder is also known as Munchausen syndrome, after the Baron von Munchausen, who was famed for his "tall tales." **Munchausen syndrome by proxy** describes the phenomenon of children in whom symptoms of illness are deliberately produced by an adult (usually a parent), so that the adult can assume the role of caretaker. These cases warrant legal intervention and protection of the child.

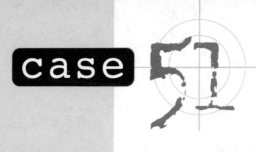

case 51

CC   A 31-year-old man presents for evaluation of recent memory problems.

HPI   Four months ago, a piece of wood fell off a high shelf at a hardware store, striking the patient on the head. According to ER records, the patient's **mental status exam was normal and the patient denied loss of consciousness.** PE was also normal without evidence of external trauma. He was monitored in the ER and discharged. However, the patient asserts that since his injury he has **intermittently forgotten** his name and where he is, leaving him unable to perform his job. He recently **filed for disability** and now **asks for a medical report documenting his deficits.**

PE   **Physical and neurologic exam normal;** on mental status exam, patient is alert and oriented to place and time; however, he has difficulty recalling his middle name; patient performs serial sevens with approximate errors; short-term memory is intact, but the patient exhibits defects in remote memories (eg, date of high school graduation, past presidents).

Labs   Lytes/CBC: normal. TFTs: normal; RPR/VDRL nonreactive; vitamin B_{12} and folate: normal.

Imaging   MRI, head: normal.

case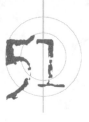

Malingering

Differential

True medical illness should always be carefully investigated and ruled out before a diagnosis of malingering is entertained. In this case, memory loss following head injury is unusual without loss of consciousness and typically involves amnesia for the accident and for the events surrounding it. Long-term memories are least likely to be affected by mild traumatic injury, and loss of orientation to person without other memory deficits seldom occurs.

Factitious disorder can be distinguished from malingering based on the nature of the incentive. In factitious disorder, the gain is motivated solely by assumption of the sick role.

Pathogenesis

Malingering involves the production or feigning of medical illness motivated by **secondary gain** (eg, financial remuneration, narcotics, housing, evading work/prison/combat). Malingering is most often seen in medicolegal cases, **disability claims**, and among prisoners and military personnel.

Management

Thorough medical and psychiatric evaluation. The patient should be given the benefit of the doubt before a diagnosis is established. Once the diagnosis is made, recommendations to the patient should be clearly and consistently articulated. The patient should be allowed to "give up" symptoms without losing dignity.

Breakout Point

> Ganser syndrome describes the phenomenon of consistently approximate (but wrong) answers to questions by patients who are exaggerating or feigning neuropsychiatric illness.

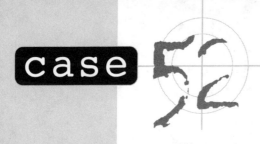

case 52

CC An 18-year-old **man** presents for an evaluation of mental status in preparation for **sex-reassignment surgery.**

HPI The patient states that as far back as he can remember, he has insisted that he is "**a woman trapped in a man's body.**" He recalls **dressing as a girl since the age of 6** and **preferring to play with his sister's toys.** His parents also report that **all of his friends were girls** and that he often found **little in common with other boys.**

PE Young-appearing male with feminine mannerisms; **normal male genitalia.**

Labs Karyotype: normal male genotype (**XY**).

case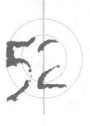

Gender Identity Disorder

Differential

Transvestic fetishism is a paraphilia that involves cross-dressing behavior for sexual excitement and typically occurs in heterosexual men. There is no insistence on cross-sex identity and no desire for sex reassignment.

Homosexuality is considered a normal variant of accepted sexual behavior and similarly does not involve insistence on cross-sex identity or desire for sex reassignment.

Pathogenesis

Gender identity disorder involves a **strong and persistent identification with the opposite gender,** typically manifesting with a **preference for cross-sex roles, dress, activities, and friends.** The precise etiology is unknown, but genetic, hormonal, neurobiologic, social learning, and psychoanalytic theories have been advanced in attempts to explain gender identity.

Epidemiology

Gender identity disorder is thought to be **more common in biological males** than in biological females.

Management

Initial management involves a thorough history, physical examination, and laboratory workup (including **karyotype analysis** in cases of ambiguous genitalia). **Psychotherapy** is useful for discussing family and other interpersonal issues regarding cross-gender preference. More specifically, psychotherapy may help the patient cope with the stress associated with cross-gender living or offer support/consultation regarding hormone therapy versus sex reassignment. **Group therapy** is useful for diminishing social withdrawal and allows participants to share ideas regarding cultural acceptance. **Sex-reassignment surgery** is reserved for adults diagnosed with true gender identity disorder.

Breakout Point

> When sex-reassignment surgery is indicated, a trial of cross-gender living for at least 1 year followed by hormone replacement is recommended before proceeding to surgery.

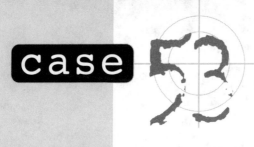

case 53

CC   A 68-year-old man is less talkative than usual while having his routine physical examination. On further questioning, the patient tells his physician that his **wife passed away 1 month ago** and that he has not felt the same since then.

HPI   The patient says he has been **sad most of the time** since his wife's death and has not been interested in his usual activities **(anhedonia).** He often **wakes up at night** and **frequently cries** when he thinks of his loss. He endorses **poor appetite** and has been skipping meals. He frequently **thinks about joining his wife** but **denies any suicidal thoughts.**

PE   Weight loss of 10 lbs since his last exam 6 months ago, otherwise physical and neurologic examinations normal.

Labs   Lytes/CBC: normal. TFTs: normal; RPR/VDRL nonreactive. UA: toxicology screen negative.

MOOD DISORDERS

case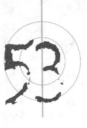

Bereavement

Differential

Major depressive disorder may be diagnosed if depressive symptoms are severe or if symptoms persist longer than currently accepted cultural norms. In bereavement, symptoms are often related to triggers regarding memories of the deceased; this differs from major depression, where symptoms tend to be chronic and recurrent without a specific trigger.

Pathogenesis

Bereavement is an **appropriate response to the death of a loved one.** If the symptoms of bereavement become severe enough or last longer than cultural norms allow, a diagnosis of a major depressive should be considered; this phenomenon may also be referred to as **complicated bereavement.** Complicated bereavement may involve prominent feelings of guilt about the loved one's death, wish to be dead, feelings of worthlessness, impairment of function, and hallucinations (excluding transiently hearing or seeing the deceased, which is a common feature of bereavement).

Management

Supportive psychotherapy is useful to help the patient with feelings of anguish, despair, and loss. If insomnia is prominent, **trazodone, zolpidem,** or **benzodiazepines** can be helpful. For those patients who go on to develop a major depressive disorder, psychotherapy and treatment with **antidepressant medications** are indicated.

Breakout Point

> Complicated bereavement has also been referred to as **pathological grief.**

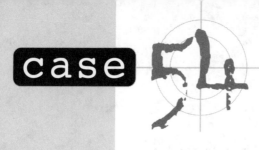

case 51

CC A **25-year-old** law student is brought to the hospital by the police after becoming agitated in his hotel lobby, shouting "I am the greatest thinker in the history of humanity!"

HPI He had suddenly traveled to Boston from Omaha a week ago with the intent of presenting his "unifying theory of everything" to "important scientists at MIT." Since checking into his hotel, he has **stayed awake for several nights without fatigue** and has **worked frantically** on his theory. He has **exceeded his credit limit** after charging several thousand dollars to his hotel room for caviar and gourmet meals. He is grasping a sheaf of crumpled papers with random numbers and symbols scrawled across them, which he claims is the result of all his work.

PE Physical and neurologic exam: normal; on mental status exam, **speech is rapid and pressured**; thought process is marked by quickly skipping from one idea to another in a **tangential** fashion (**flight of ideas**) and an inability to provide simple and direct answers to questions, instead embarking on extended soliloquies that seem to be circle around the answer (**circumstantiality**); patient also endorses **racing thoughts**.

Labs Lytes/CBC: normal. TFTs: normal; RPR/VDRL nonreactive. UA: toxicology screen negative.

Imaging CT, head: normal.

MOOD DISORDERS

107

case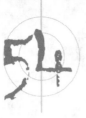

Bipolar I Disorder

Differential

Bipolar II disorder is characterized by **hypomanic** and depressive episodes; hypomania requires only 4 days of symptoms with no impairment of social or occupational functioning.

Major depressive disorder lacks a history of mania or hypomania.

Substance-induced mood disorder/acute intoxication from cocaine, amphetamines, or PCP may cause agitation, pressured speech, and psychosis. Urine toxicology screen and thorough history are essential to accurate diagnosis.

Hyperthyroidism can mimic the signs and symptoms of mania. TFTs should be checked in patients presenting with mania.

Pathogenesis

Bipolar I disorder is defined by episodes of both elevated and depressed mood with the occurrence of **at least one manic episode** featuring **1 week or more** of symptoms including **grandiosity, decreased need for sleep,** pressured speech, flight of ideas, **distractibility, increased goal-oriented activity,** and **injudicious impulsive behavior** (eg, spending sprees, sexual promiscuity, gambling). Symptoms **must cause marked impairment in occupational or social functioning.** Bipolar disorder has not yet been linked to a specific neurotransmitter system, although twin studies indicate a **strong genetic component.**

Epidemiology

Males and females are equally affected; **average age at onset is 20 years.**

Complications

Approximately 90% of individuals who suffer a manic episode will have **future recurrences** if left untreated. Future episodes will likely occur with greater frequency, intensity, and less dependence on external stimuli for initiation. Patients with bipolar illness carry a **significant risk of suicide.**

Management

Mood stabilizers and **neuroleptics** (olanzapine) constitute first-line pharmacotherapy. Adverse effects of mood stabilizers vary and require monitoring; **lithium** may cause hypothyroidism, tremor, nephrogenic diabetes insipidus, arrhythmias, and fetal cardiac defects (**Ebstein anomaly**). **Valproic acid** (Depakote, Depakene) may cause **hepatotoxicity,** pancreatitis, tremor, thrombocytopenia, and fetal neural tube defects. Other mood stabilizers include carbamazepine (Tegretol), oxcarbazepine (Trileptal), and lamotrigine (Lamictal). For concurrent agitation or psychosis, add **benzodiazepines** or **neuroleptics** to mood stabilizers. **Antidepressants** should first be titrated to therapeutic levels as "unopposed" antidepressants may precipitate mania. **ECT** can be beneficial in severe or refractory cases of mania or depression.

Breakout Point

Signs and Symptoms of Mania (DIG FAST)			
Distractibility	**G**randiosity	**A**ctivity (increased)	**T**alkativeness
Indiscretion	**F**light of Ideas	**S**leep Deficit	

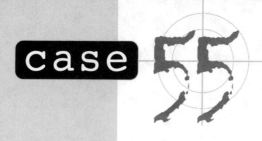

case

CC A 33-year-old divorced woman returns to her primary care physician for follow-up after starting fluoxetine 4 weeks ago for **depressed mood**.

HPI She had initially presented with 4 months of increasing **fatigue, difficulty concentrating, weight gain**, and **suicidal thoughts**. She now reports little change in her symptoms since starting her antidepressant. She spends most of the day sleeping in bed and finds that she does not enjoy her usual activities **(anhedonia)**.

PE VS: **bradycardia** (HR 56); hypotension (BP 80/40). PE: **skin coarse and dry; diminished reflexes throughout;** on mental status exam, **speech is slowed;** patient has **impairment of short-term memory and attention** as evidenced by recalling only one of three objects after 5 minutes and difficulty counting backwards by sevens.

Labs **Elevated TSH** (20 μIU/mL); **low total T$_4$** (2.2 μg/dL); elevated lipids.

case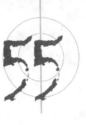

Mood Disorder Due to a General Medical Condition

Differential | **Major depressive disorder** cannot be diagnosed until an underlying medical condition is either ruled out or adequately treated.

Pathogenesis | **Mood disorder due to a general medical condition** is diagnosed if the mood disturbance (either depressive, manic, or mixed) is the **direct physiologic consequence** of a medical condition. Common examples include **hypothyroidism,** cerebrovascular disease, MS, cancer (especially pancreatic and CNS), Cushing disease, lupus, Addison disease, sleep apnea, and Parkinson disease.

Management | **Treatment of the underlying medical condition** should take priority; concurrent antidepressant therapy may be indicated if the depression is severe and slow to respond. In this case, hypothyroidism should be treated with thyroxine.

Breakout Point |

> Thyroxine is sometimes used as an adjunct to antidepressants in the treatment of medication-resistant major depression.

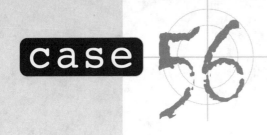

case 56

CC A 70-year-old **woman** is seen by her internist for **weight loss, fatigue,** and **insomnia** over **at least the past 2 weeks.**

HPI The patient says that she has not felt the same since she moved into a nursing home due to her failing health. She feels that since all her friends have passed away, she does not have anything to live for and **thinks about death frequently** (morbid preoccupations). She denies **suicidal thoughts** but feels that she would be better off dead. She also reports **poor concentration** and **trouble remembering** things. She **no longer takes pleasure** in her hobbies **(anhedonia)**, has "**no appetite** for food," and **feels worthless** and **guilty** regarding past relationships.

PE VS: normal. PE: mental status exam significant for **depressed mood, psychomotor retardation,** and **impaired short-term memory.**

Labs Lytes/CBC: normal. TFTs: normal; RPR nonreactive.

case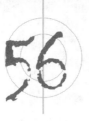

Major Depressive Disorder

Differential

Mood disorder due to a general medical condition requires a mood disturbance that is the direct physiologic consequence of a medical condition.

Dysthymia involves symptoms of depression lasting at least 2 years and does not meet the full criteria for major depressive disorder.

Adjustment disorder with depressed mood requires an identifiable psychosocial stressor and symptoms do not meet the full criteria for major depressive disorder.

Substance-induced mood disorder should be considered when depressive symptoms occur within 1 month of substance intoxication or withdrawal.

Bereavement is diagnosed when symptoms of a major depressive episode occur after the loss of a loved one. Symptoms that last more than 2 months and involve suicidal ideations, morbid preoccupations, or psychosis warrant a diagnosis of major depression.

Pathogenesis

A diagnosis of major depressive disorder requires depressed mood plus **at least four of the SIGECAPS symptoms** (Breakout Point box) persisting **for at least 2 weeks.** Major depressive disorder is likely due to complex interactions of genetic, psychosocial, and neurobiologic factors. The **serotonergic** and **noradrenergic** systems have been strongly implicated in depression. Antidepressants work by affecting transmission in either or both of these systems.

Epidemiology

Females are affected more often than males by a ratio of 2 to 1; **lifetime prevalence is about 10%.**

Management

Psychotherapy and pharmacotherapy are both efficacious for depressive syndromes, especially when employed concurrently. **SSRIs** (fluoxetine [Prozac], sertraline [Zoloft], paroxetine [Paxil], citalopram [Celexa], and escitalopram [Lexapro]) **have become first-line pharmacologic agents.** Other first-line agents include **bupropion** (Wellbutrin), **venlafaxine** (Effexor), **duloxetine** (Cymbalta), and mirtazapine (Remeron). **TCAs** are now considered to be second-line agents because of their side effect profile and **potential for fatal overdose.** Depression that fails to resolve with multiple 6-week trials of the above therapies may warrant consideration of pharmacologic **augmentation strategies** (including lithium carbonate and thyroid hormone), **MAO inhibitors,** or **ECT.**

Breakout Point

Symptoms of Major Depression (SIG E CAPS)	
Sleep Disturbance	Concentration Decrease
Interests Decreased (anhedonia)	Appetite Disturbance
Guilt	Psychomotor Agitation or Retardation
Energy Decreased	Suicidality or Preoccupation with Death
Diagnosis requires at least five symptoms for more than 2 weeks.	

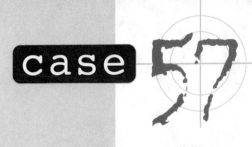

case 57

CC A 26-year-old **unmarried woman** presents to her primary care physician complaining of **feeling sad and hopeless.** She states that she has felt persistently depressed for "**at least the last 2 years.**"

HPI The patient reports feeling **fatigued** at times and having poor self-esteem. However, she **denies any significant disturbance in sleep or appetite.** She **denies suicidal or homicidal ideation** and denies morbid ruminations. During the past 2 years, she has never been free of symptoms for more than 2 months at a time.

PE Physical and neurologic exams normal.

Labs Lytes/CBC: normal. TFTs: normal; RPR/VDRL nonreactive. UA: toxicology screen negative.

case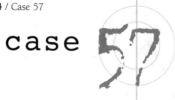

Dysthymic Disorder

Differential

Major depressive disorder can be distinguished from dysthymia by the number of criteria that are met for a major depressive episode and the duration of symptoms.

Adjustment disorder with depressed mood involves symptoms that are due to an identifiable psychosocial stressor within the 3 months prior to the onset of symptoms.

Mood disorder due to a general medical condition must involve a direct physiologic relationship between the illness and mood.

Pathogenesis

A diagnosis of dysthymic disorder requires persistent depressed mood, **occurring on more days than not,** for **at least 2 years,** along with at least two of the following symptoms: appetite disturbance, sleep disturbance, low energy, poor self-esteem, poor concentration, or feelings of hopelessness.

Although no clear etiology has been identified, psychological models and neurobiologic mechanisms have been implicated in dysthymic disorder. A major depressive episode may superimpose itself on dysthymic disorder, a phenomenon known as **"double depression."** Patients are at increased risk for other **comorbid psychiatric illnesses,** especially substance abuse.

Management

The treatment of dysthymia mirrors that of major depression. **Psychotherapy** and pharmacotherapy are effective. Successful pharmacologic agents include **SSRIs, bupropion, venlafaxine, duloxetine, TCAs,** and **MAO inhibitors** (phenelzine, tranylcypromine).

Breakout Point

Symptoms of Dysthymia (Self-Esteem ACHES)
Self-Esteem (decreased)
Appetite (increased or decreased)
Concentration (decreased)
Hopelessness
Energy (decreased)
Sleep (increased or decreased)

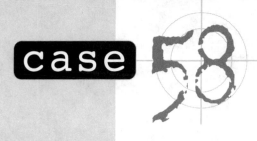

case 58

CC   A 23-year-old **woman** graduate student is brought to her psychiatrist's office by her roommate complaining that she has been **up all night working** noisily on "a million different projects."

HPI   The patient has a **history of major depressive episodes** but had tapered off her antidepressant and had a **normal range of mood** (euthymia) over the past year. Her roommate noticed that about **4 days** ago the patient became **markedly more active** in her graduate school research, working **all night**, talking about her **superiority to the others** in her program, and **chatting familiarly** with strangers. Despite this, the patient had **not acted bizarrely** and was **meeting all her deadlines for school.**

PE   VS and PE are normal. Mental status exam reveals a markedly **talkative woman** whose thought processes **quickly jump from one idea to another.** She does state that her **thoughts are moving fast.** She **does not display any bizarre behavior** and **denies any auditory or visual hallucinations.**

Labs   Toxicology screens: negative; TFTs: within normal limits.

case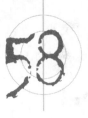

Bipolar II Disorder

Differential

Bipolar I disorder can be differentiated from bipolar II disorder by the presence of mania. The lack of significant impairment in social or occupational functioning and the absence of psychosis or symptoms that necessitate psychiatric hospitalization **differentiate hypomania from mania.**

Substance-induced mood disorder/acute intoxication from cocaine, amphetamines, or other stimulants may mimic hypomania. Urine toxicology screen and thorough history are essential to accurate diagnosis.

Pathogenesis

A diagnosis of **bipolar II disorder** is made when there is a history of **at least one major depressive episode** and **at least one hypomanic episode.** *There cannot be any history of mania.* Hypomania is characterized by the DSM-IV as an unusually elevated, expansive, or irritable mood lasting at least 4 days. Hypomania is diagnosed if **three or more** the following criteria are met **(four are needed if the mood is only irritable)**: inflated self-esteem or **grandiosity, decreased need for sleep, more talkative** than usual or pressure to keep talking, **flight of ideas** or feeling that **thoughts are racing, distractibility, increase in goal-directed activity,** and **excessive involvement in pleasurable activities** with high risk of problematic outcomes (spending, sex, haphazard investing).

Management

Bipolar II disorder is usually managed with **mood stabilizers** (lithium, valproate), and, if needed, **antidepressants.** Care should be used when prescribing antidepressants to patients with bipolar II disorder, because they can precipitate hypomania or mania.

Breakout Point

> The phenomenon of an antidepressant inducing mania or hypomania is often referred to as **"manic switch."** Symptoms that appear hypomanic but are caused by an antidepressant treatment do not meet criteria for a diagnosis of bipolar II disorder.

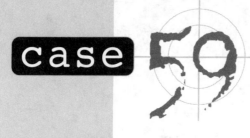

case 59

CC   A 39-year-old woman presents for an evaluation of ongoing depressed mood. She notes that she **regularly has a worsening of her mood in the fall.** She states, "I just want to hibernate when October comes."

HPI   She has a **4-year history of a distinct worsening of mood starting in the fall and continuing through the winter.** She recalls that all her life she felt "poorly in the winter" but thought she "just didn't like the cold." Over the past years the yearly mood change had become distinct and has affected her daily functioning. She endorses **fatigue** that prevents her from getting her work done, **eating "comfort foods,"** and **sleeping "until the afternoon if I can."** She reports frequent crying and **does not enjoy her hobbies such as knitting and needlepoint.** Her poor mood lasts "pretty much **until spring, then it seems to lift.**"

PE   Mental status exam is remarkable for a tearful, overweight woman, slumped in her chair.

Labs   TSH: normal; CBC: normal.

MOOD DISORDERS

117

case 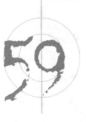 59

Seasonal Affective Disorder (SAD)

Differential

The differential diagnosis for SAD is similar to that for major depressive disorder and includes dysthymic disorder, adjustment disorder with depressed mood, substance-induced mood disorder, and mood disorder due to a general medical condition. Careful history is vital to an accurate diagnosis.

Pathogenesis

SAD is classified in the DSM-IV as a **"seasonal pattern specifier" for the pattern of major depressive episodes in bipolar I, bipolar II, or major depressive disorder.** "Seasonal pattern specifier" requires that a major depressive episode occur at a **particular time of the year.** Full remissions or mood shifts also occur with a yearly pattern. This pattern of mood changes must have occurred for **at least the past 2 years.** In addition, when looking back over the lifespan, seasonal depressions should outnumber any nonseasonal depressions. Seasonal depression is frequently characterized by **low energy, overeating, hypersomnia, weight gain,** and **carbohydrate craving.**

Epidemiology

SAD occurs more commonly in women and is more often found at higher latitudes.

Management

SAD, like major depressive episodes, may be treated with **antidepressants such as SSRIs. Light therapy (phototherapy) is also common.** In patients with a history of mania or hypomania, caution should be taken when prescribing phototherapy because like antidepressant medications, this treatment may promote an episode of mania or hypomania.

Breakout Point

> The recommended exposure for phototherapy is at least 30 minutes daily to 10,000 lux light.

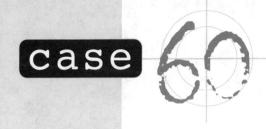

case 60

CC A 31-year woman **3 weeks' postpartum** from the birth of her first child presents to her obstetrician's office complaining that **"I am not enjoying my baby or anything else."**

HPI **Two weeks after giving birth she started to feel depressed and anxious.** She states that she had felt "overwhelmed and sad" after the birth of her son, and now that her husband has returned to work, she also feels alone and isolated. She reports continually **worrying that she would somehow harm the infant,** and is fearful that she is "not doing things right." **She firmly denies any thoughts of harming her infant or herself,** but she thinks of herself as "severely deficient in mothering skills." She is having **trouble sleeping** even aside from the breast-feeding schedule, and her **energy is consistently low.** Her husband is concerned that she **is frequently tearful and not eating enough.** She concluded, "maternity leave is not what I thought it would be."

PE The patient is seen with her infant, and she is very attentive to him. She is tearful when describing her mood.

Labs TSH: normal.

case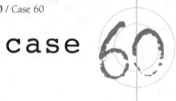

Postpartum Depression

Differential

Baby blues affects many (>50%) of women and shares some of the features of postpartum depression but occurs in the first days after delivery, is self limited (days to weeks), and does not impair functioning.

Postpartum psychosis is characterized by symptoms such as delusions and hallucinations and is a **psychiatric emergency** because the mother is at increased risk to harm both her infant and herself.

Pathogenesis

Postpartum depression shares the characteristics of a major depressive episode. Postpartum depression may have an onset within days of delivery, although it **usually occurs several weeks after giving birth** and may last for months if untreated. The risk of postpartum mood disorder is increased if the woman has a history of nonpostpartum or postpartum mood episodes. **Symptoms of anxiety** may accompany the depressive symptoms.

Management

Early detection is vital for timely treatment of postpartum depression. Obstetricians should routinely screen for current symptoms, personal history, and family history of depression throughout pregnancy. SSRIs or another antidepressant and/or psychotherapy are treatments of choice for postpartum depression. If a woman is breast-feeding, the **risks and benefits of psychopharmacologic treatment** must be considered for both the mother and the infant.

Breakout Point

> The diagnosis of postpartum depression is confounded by the fact that women typically have lower energy, poor concentration, interrupted sleep, and changes in eating patterns after giving birth.

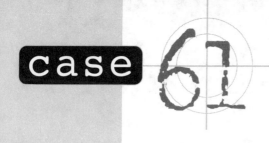

case 62

CC   A 25-year-old **man** is brought to the ER following an automobile accident.

HPI   The police report that the patient deliberately cut off another vehicle. The patient has previously been imprisoned for vehicular assault. He demonstrates **a lack of remorse** and a **disregard for the safety of others,** noting that "the jackass was driving too slowly and deserved what he got." He has a long history of **impulsive behavior, disorderly and aggressive conduct,** and was **diagnosed with conduct disorder before the age of 15 years.**

PE   Minor abrasion to forehead, multiple tattoos; mental status exam within normal limits.

Labs   Urine toxicology negative.

Imaging   XR, cervical and thoracic spine: unremarkable. CT, head (noncontrast): negative.

PERSONALITY DISORDERS

case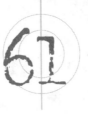

Antisocial Personality Disorder

Differential

Narcissistic personality disorder may feature the sense of entitlement and desire for admiration associated with antisocial personality disorder; however, narcissistic personality disorder typically lacks impulsivity, overt aggression, and disregard for the rights of others.

Conduct disorder is diagnosed if the patient is younger than 18 years old. Evidence of conduct disorder prior to the age of 15 is one of the diagnostic criteria of antisocial personality disorder.

Substance abuse commonly coexists with antisocial personality disorder. However, antisocial personality disorder reflects a persistent maladaptive pattern of behavior that is present in the absence of any substance use. Toxicology screen and clinical history can help establish the temporal relationship of behavior and substance use.

Head injury, especially to the frontal lobes, can result in the impulsive and reckless behavior associated with antisocial personality disorder. In fact, it has been postulated that many cases of antisocial personality disorder are the direct result of head injury.

Pathogenesis

Antisocial personality disorder involves an inflexible, maladaptive, and pervasive pattern of disregard for the rights of others. The etiology of antisocial personality disorder is multifactorial, likely involving an interaction between genetic predisposition and environmental stressors. Risk factors include an **unstable home environment** and **substance abuse.**

Epidemiology

Males are **affected more than females,** with a prevalence of 5% in men and 1% in women.

Management

Antisocial personality disorder is sometimes amenable to long-term psychotherapy with strict limit-setting. Pharmacotherapy is reserved for comorbid illnesses. Antisocial personalities frequently attempt to destroy, exploit, or avoid therapeutic relationships. Groups are helpful in that peer interaction minimizes issues with authority.

Breakout Point

Diagnostic Criteria for Antisocial Personality Disorder (CORRUPT)
Cannot Follow Law
Obligations Ignored
Remorseless
Reckless
Underhanded
Planning Deficit
Temper
At least three are required for diagnosis.

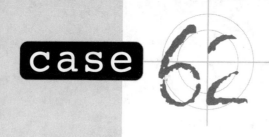

case 62

CC   A 23-year-old **woman** is brought to the ER after deliberately **cutting herself** on the left forearm.

HPI   She endorses cutting herself because her boyfriend went to dinner with a female classmate. The patient has a long history of **impulsive behavior** (including sexual promiscuity and substance abuse) and **self-mutilating behavior** in previous relationships, apparently as **attempts to avoid feeling abandoned**. Her **relationships have been stormy, intense, and unstable.** She has been hospitalized for overdoses and self-mutilation, and reports that cutting relieves her **chronic feelings of emptiness.** She appears **affectively unstable,** becoming **inappropriately angry** when examined by the chief resident and laughing pleasantly shortly thereafter while her blood is drawn.

PE   Three superficial lacerations distal to the left antecubital fossa; well-healed scars on both arms.

Imaging   Cutting of arms.

case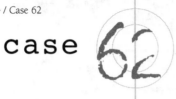

Borderline Personality Disorder

Differential

Mood disorders (eg, major depressive disorder, bipolar disorder) often occur comorbidly with borderline personality disorder, and distinguishing them may be difficult. Borderline personality disorder is characterized by a consistent maladaptive pattern of relationships and self-image beginning in adolescence, whereas mood disorders typically are not characterized by the consistent pattern of stress-related paranoid ideations, dissociative experiences, or self-damaging impulsive behaviors found in borderline personality disorder.

Histrionic personality disorder may manifest with affective instability and need for attention; however, the self-destructive behaviors, dissociative experiences, and feelings of emptiness associated with borderline personality disorder are lacking.

Pathogenesis

Borderline personality disorder involves a **persistent and pervasive pattern** of **difficulties with relationships, affect management,** and **impulsive self-harming behaviors.** No single etiology has been identified for borderline personality disorder; however, a biopsychosocial model involving the interaction between genetic and developmental experiences has been implicated. Notably, patients with borderline personality disorder frequently have a **history of physical and/or sexual abuse** during their formative years.

Management

Careful evaluation for comorbid axis I disorders (including PTSD, mood disorders, psychotic disorders, and substance abuse disorders) should be undertaken during any assessment. **Dialectical behavioral therapy,** a modified version of CBT focused on minimizing self-harming behavior, is currently the most effective treatment for borderline personality disorder. Pharmacotherapeutic approaches target symptoms of mood instability, anxiety, impulsive behavior, and "micropsychotic" episodes, often using combinations of antidepressants, mood stabilizers, and neuroleptics.

Breakout Point

Diagnostic Criteria for Borderline Personality Disorder (IMPULSIVE) at Least Five Are Required for Diagnosis
Impulsive
Moody
Paranoia or Dissociation under Stress
Unstable Self-Image
Labile Intense Relationships
Suicidal Acts
Inappropriate Anger
Vulnerability to Abandonment
Emptiness (chronic feelings of)
At least five are required for diagnosis.

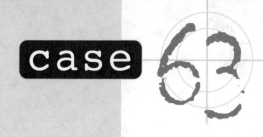

CC A 42-year-old man is referred for a psychiatric evaluation by his employer to obtain a higher-level security clearance.

HPI The patient works as a computer engineer for a nuclear submarine manufacturer that contracts with the government. He has **never had any close friends** and **rarely interacts with others** at work. He states that he is content with his work and has **little interest in social contacts or romantic relationships.** Given the choice, the patient prefers **solitary activities** to keep busy. He has no prior history of mood disturbance, cognitive deficits, or psychotic symptoms.

PE On mental status exam, **affect** is **flat and detached** and mood is euthymic; no evidence of delusions, hallucinations, or disorganized thought processes; attention, concentration, memory, and abstract thinking are intact.

PERSONALITY DISORDERS

case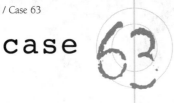

Schizoid Personality Disorder

Differential

Avoidant personality disorder can be distinguished from schizoid personality disorder by the desire for social interactions. In avoidant personality disorder, the patient seeks social intimacy but fears rejection and feelings of inadequacy, whereas in schizoid personality disorder, no interaction is desired.

Schizotypal personality disorder involves perceptual distortions (eg, odd thinking, ideas of reference, illusions), eccentric appearance, and excessive social anxiety.

Pathogenesis

Schizoid personality disorder involves a persistent and pervasive pattern of detachment from social relationships and restricted emotion. Genetic and psychosocial models have been proposed for causes of schizoid personality disorder, but little evidence exists for either.

Management

Patients with schizoid personality disorder infrequently self-present to psychiatrists because of their **aloof and detached** nature. Furthermore, many individuals with schizoid personality disorder are able to **perform well at jobs that do not require significant social interaction,** keeping them from referral. Although they do not have significant social relationships, **they do not perceive this as a deficit,** and thus they do not seek treatment.

Breakout Point

Personality disorders are divided into three clusters:

Cluster A: Paranoid, Schizoid, Schizotypal
Cluster B: Antisocial, Borderline, Histrionic, Narcissistic
Cluster C: Avoidant, Dependent, Obsessive-Compulsive

The three clusters can be broadly summarized by the **"three Ws": W**eird (cluster A), **W**ild (cluster B), and **W**impy (cluster C).

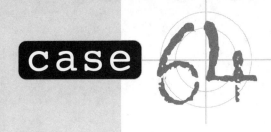

case 64

CC   A 38-year-old unemployed man is referred to the psychiatry clinic by his new day program.

HPI   The patient recently began attending a local day program after his parents insisted that he participate in a daytime activity outside of the home. Previously, he spent his days at home, where he lives with his parents who support him financially. He has had various part-time jobs in the past but found jobs difficult to maintain because he believed his coworkers were jealous of his **special abilities.** He **believes he has a gift** for journalism and produces a two-page weekly newspaper that enumerates his **odd opinions** regarding government misuse of tax money. He has **no friends,** stating that other people just plagiarize his writing. Sometimes he experiences **unusual bodily sensations,** which he calls an "other-worldly feeling." These sensations indicate to him he is about to have a journalistic inspiration. He has never been hospitalized, diagnosed with any psychiatric illness, or received any psychiatric medications.

PE   On mental status exam, he is polite but somewhat **guarded,** frequently asking "why do you need to know that?" He asks if the interview is being recorded. There is no evidence of hallucinations, bizarre delusions, or disorganization of thought.

case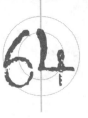

Schizotypal Personality Disorder

Differential

Schizoid personality disorder presents with similar social isolation but lacks the cognitive distortions and odd behavior seen in schizotypal personality disorder. **Schizophrenia** can be distinguished from schizotypal personality disorder by the presence of bizarre delusions, hallucinations, extreme disorganization, or severe negative symptoms.

Pathogenesis

Schizotypal personality disorder describes a pervasive pattern of deficits in interpersonal and social functioning, accompanied by markedly eccentric behavior and cognitive or perceptual distortions.

Epidemiology

It affects approximately 3% of the population and occurs slightly more frequently in males. Patients with schizotypal personality disorder have an increased likelihood of having a close relative with schizophrenia.

Management

Patients with schizotypal personality disorder frequently are paranoid of treaters and do not often present voluntarily for assessment. It is important to focus on building an alliance in the initial stages of treatment. Neuroleptics may be helpful for treatment of paranoia. Anxiolytics may help patients tolerate social interactions.

Breakout Point

> Patients with schizotypal personality disorder may have unusual or odd beliefs. It is important to take great care to avoid belittling or ridiculing these beliefs in order to maintain a workable therapeutic relationship.

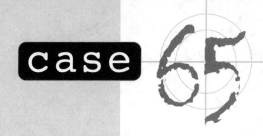

case 65

CC
A 43-year-old business manager visits a psychiatrist for the first time, upset that his third wife has mentioned divorce, asking "what is **her** problem?"

HPI
He arrives 25 minutes late and, calling the psychiatrist by his first name, says: "Listen, Bill, I had a really important meeting to attend, but of course we still have the full hour, right?" He explains that his marriage is failing because he thinks his wife is jealous of his business success and good looks. He describes similar problems with his first two wives. He **brags** about the size of his corporation, explaining that he is the "heart and soul" of the company, but he complains that others are jealous of his "special way with people" and have "weaseled their way ahead of me." When asked if there is anything he would like to change about himself, the man replies: "Bill, I just want to be appreciated for how hard I work and have my wife stop being so difficult."

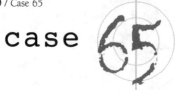

case

Narcissistic Personality Disorder

Differential

Antisocial personality disorder features impulsive behavior and reckless disregard for safety not seen in narcissistic personality disorder.

Borderline personality disorder differs in that people with narcissistic personality disorder have a more stable (although inflated) sense of self and do not fear abandonment.

Bipolar disorder with mania or hypomania may feature prominent grandiosity, a thorough history, including an assessment for the signs and symptoms of mania, is vital to accurate diagnosis. As with other personality disorders, those with narcissistic personality disorder may also have comorbid axis I psychopathology.

Pathogenesis

Narcissistic personality disorder comprises a pervasive pattern of **grandiosity, need for admiration,** and **lack of empathy.** Five out of nine diagnostic criteria are required (Breakout Point box). Children of parents with narcissistic personality disorder may be at increased risk for developing the disorder, with their parents instilling grandiosity, entitlement, and lack of empathy.

Management

The mainstay of treatment is **individual psychotherapy;** however, some advocate group psychotherapy so that individuals can learn how to share with others and be more empathic. Narcissistic personality disorder is **difficult to treat,** because the individual often fails to acknowledge that the problem rests within himself or herself and not with others.

Breakout Point

Diagnostics Criteria for Narcissistic Personality Disorder (GRANDIOSE)
Grandiose
Requires Attention
Arrogant
Need to be Special
Dreams of Success and Power
Interpersonally Exploitative
Others (unable to recognize feelings/needs of)
Sense of Entitlement
Envious
At least five required for diagnosis.

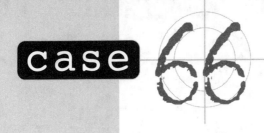

case 66

CC A 41-year-old woman seeking psychotherapy for the first time presents with the complaint, "I can't keep a boyfriend for more than 3 months; I'll never get married!"

HPI She cannot understand why, as the **"life of the party,"** she is **able to make, but not keep, friends.** She has dated many men, but they often "disappear" or "stop calling" for reasons unknown to her. She **tearfully** notes that after her "nose job" she thought she would be able to "meet someone special." She goes on to state **laughingly** that she realizes she is **"way too interesting"** to care about what other people do. She **dramatically** recalls her "terrible upbringing" as a "wealthy, forgotten child" and wonders if the therapist finds her "difficult to figure out." At the end of the session, she notes that she has **already developed a "close connection" with her therapist** and wonders if they could meet twice a week, perhaps at her favorite coffee shop.

PE On exam the patient is dressed in **a low-cut bright purple sweater** and **wearing large rhinestone earrings.** When speaking, she waves her arms and intermittently shifts her chair closer to her therapist.

case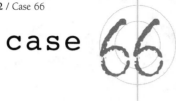

Histrionic Personality Disorder

Differential | **Borderline personality disorder** also manifests with affective instability and need for attention; however, it also features prominent disturbance of identity, self-destructive behaviors, dissociative experiences, and feelings of emptiness.

Narcissistic personality disorder also features a pronounced need for attention, but typically also includes grandiosity, arrogance, exploitiveness, and jealousy.

Pathogenesis | Histrionic personality disorder is a **cluster B personality disorder** characterized by a **repetitive pattern of dramatic and attention-seeking behavior**. The DSM-IV requires at least **five of a possible eight** diagnostic criteria (Breakout Point box) for a diagnosis of histrionic personality disorder.

Management | **Psychotherapy is the treatment of choice** for histrionic personality disorder, but medications may be used for symptoms, such as anxiety and depression, that may complicate the clinical picture.

Breakout Point

Diagnostic Criteria for Histrionic Personality Disorder (PRAISE ME)

Provocative or Seductive Behavior
Relationships (considered more intimate than they actually are)
Attention (must be at center of)
Influenced Easily
Speech (impressionistic style, lacking in detail)
Emotions (shifting and shallow)
Make-Up (physical appearance used to draw attention to self)
Exaggerated Dramatic Expression of Emotions
At least five are required for diagnosis.

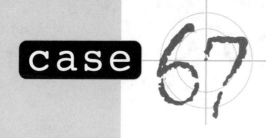

case 67

CC A 26-year-old police officer is brought to the ER by his colleagues, who are concerned about a recent **change in his behavior.**

HPI For **2 weeks** he has been convinced that the other officers are trying to frame him. He thinks they want to kick him off the force because "they can read my dirty thoughts." His wife confirms this history, adding that he has had a "short fuse" lately and has seemed paranoid, insisting that the blinds on the windows be kept closed. She also notes that he has been **suspicious** of his coworkers since having been passed up for a promotion **less than 1 month ago.**

PE Neurologic and physical exams normal; on mental status exam, patient acts bizarrely and answers questions in a loose and disorganized fashion.

Labs UA: toxicology screen negative.

Imaging MRI, head: normal.

case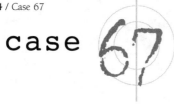

Brief Psychotic Disorder

Differential

Schizophreniform disorder is diagnosed when psychotic symptoms (hallucinations, delusions, disorganized behavior) are present for 1 to 6 months.

Schizophrenia should be diagnosed when psychosis persists for more than 6 months.

Delusional disorder has symptoms that are present for at least 1 month, but the presentation is limited to a fixed and well-circumscribed delusion without other prominent psychotic symptoms such as hallucinations, bizarre delusions, or grossly disorganized speech/behavior.

Pathogenesis

Brief psychotic disorder is diagnosed when symptoms of delusions, hallucinations, disorganized speech, or disorganized behavior persist for more than 1 day but less than 1 month. Fifty to eighty percent of patients diagnosed with brief psychotic disorder never have another psychotic episode. Brief psychotic disorder is associated with an increased risk of suicide.

Management

Treatment is similar to that of psychotic episodes associated with chronic psychotic illness. **Neuroleptics** (haloperidol, perphenazine, chlorpromazine, risperidone, olanzapine, quetiapine) are used to treat psychotic and agitated behavior. **Benzodiazepines** may also be used to treat anxiety and severe agitation. Supportive psychotherapy is a useful adjunct in the presence of precipitating stressors.

Breakout Point

> Brief psychotic disorder, schizophreniform disorder, and schizophrenia exist on a chronological spectrum, with changes in diagnosis occurring after 1 and 6 months of persistent symptoms.

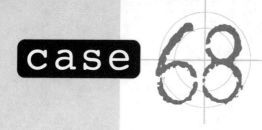

case 68

CC A 38-year-old man presents to a local police station complaining that the **Federal Bureau of Investigation (FBI) has been following him** unjustly for **at least 1 month.**

HPI The patient believes that the FBI has placed him on surveillance since his visit to the White House earlier this year. Since then, he believes that the FBI has expanded its coverage of him, listening to his phone conversations and eavesdropping on his social interactions. He is successfully employed, and his **functioning has not been significantly impaired by the distractions.** He does not feel particularly threatened but requests that the police intervene on his behalf.

PE Physical and neurologic exams normal.

Labs Lytes/CBC: normal. Toxicology screens negative.

Imaging CT, head: normal.

case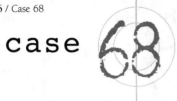

Delusional Disorder

Differential

Delusional disorder, erotomanic type is characterized by the patient's false belief that another person is in love with them.

Delusional disorder, grandiose type is characterized by delusions of exaggerated power, knowledge, wealth, or relationship to famous figures.

Delusional disorder, jealous type involves the delusion that the patient's partner is unfaithful.

Delusional disorder, somatic type involves the delusion that the patient has a physical defect or medical condition.

Delusional disorder, mixed type is used to describe a delusional disorder that involves more than one of the above types.

Paranoid personality disorder is characterized by pervasive distrust that extends into most relationships and is not encompassed by a single delusion.

Chronic paranoid schizophrenia and other psychotic disorders involve disorganization of behavior and speech, negative symptoms, hallucinations, and bizarre delusions.

Major depressive disorder with psychotic features involves mood-congruent delusions occurring concurrently with a major mood disturbance.

Pathogenesis

Delusional disorder is marked by a **powerful, well-circumscribed delusion without other signs or symptoms of psychosis.** Delusions are **nonbizarre in quality** in that they address situations that occur in everyday life (eg, having an illness or a cheating spouse). The etiology of delusional disorder is unknown, and its course tends to be **chronic** and **unremitting.** The **persecutory type** of delusional disorder is the **most common.**

Epidemiology

Delusional disorder is **rare;** prevalence has been estimated at 0.05%.

Management

Psychotherapy may offer some benefit. Pharmacotherapy with pimozide (Orap) or another neuroleptic may be helpful, although **most cases of delusional disorder are refractory to treatment.** Always carefully assess the patient's risk of endangering himself or others.

Breakout Point

> The delusion of being loved or romantically pursued by another person, usually of higher status, is also known as DeClerembault syndrome.

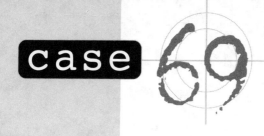

case 69

CC A **22-year-old** man is brought to the hospital by his parents secondary to increasingly **bizarre behavior** over the past **6 months.**

HPI The patient's parents relate a normal developmental history but note that their son has always kept to himself and had **few friends** while growing up. Last year, during his junior year of college, his grades began to deteriorate and he took a semester off. Since then, his parents report that he **talks to himself, fails to maintain appropriate hygiene, expresses no emotions,** and shows no interest in going back to school.

PE Physical exam normal; on mental status exam, patient reports **hearing multiple voices** that frequently comment on his actions; he also reports **receiving messages from God** through his television; **affect is flat** and **thought process is difficult to follow.**

Labs Lytes/CBC: normal. BUN and creatinine: normal; TFTs: normal; RPR nonreactive. UA: toxicology screen negative.

Imaging CT, head, for schizophrenia.

case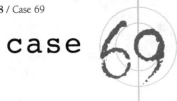

Schizophrenia

Differential

Substance-induced psychotic disorders may be distinguished from schizophrenia via a careful history to establish a temporal relationship of symptoms to drug use, coupled with urine toxicology and physical exam.

Schizoaffective disorder is diagnosed when the criteria for both schizophrenia and an affective disorder are met, with at least a 2-week period of psychotic symptoms in the absence of mood disturbance.

Schizophreniform disorder is diagnosed when criteria for schizophrenia are present for more than 1 month but less than 6 months; it may progress to schizophrenia.

Delusional disorder may be distinguished by the nonbizarre nature of the delusion and the absence of auditory hallucinations or disorganized behavior.

Brief psychotic disorder involves psychotic symptoms present for more than 1 day but but less than 1 month.

Pathogenesis

A diagnosis of schizophrenia requires **at least 6 months** of functional disturbance, including at least 1 month of two or more of the following: positive symptoms (delusions, hallucinations, disorganized speech, disorganized/catatonic behavior) or negative symptoms (**flattening of affect, poverty of speech, poor hygiene, or amotivation**). Although the exact mechanism of schizophrenia is unknown, genetic and neurodevelopmental factors likely play a central role. The **dopamine hypothesis** posits that symptoms are the result of **increased dopaminergic transmission in the mesolimbic area,** but other neurotransmitter systems have been implicated (GABA, glutamate, NMDA, and serotonin).

Epidemiology

Prevalence is 1%; males and females are equally affected. Average age of **onset is younger in males** (early 20s) than females (mid to late 20s).

Complications

Suicide is the leading cause of mortality in this population (15% of patients), with 50% of patients making attempts.

Management

Occupational and social skills training for the patient as well as family education and therapy are helpful. First-line pharmacologic management should consist of an **atypical** or a **typical neuroleptic. Atypical neuroleptics** (clozapine, risperidone, olanzapine, quetiapine, ziprasidone, aripiprazole) have **fewer extrapyramidal side effects,** whereas the efficacy of typical neuroleptics (chlorpromazine, perphenazine, fluphenazine, haloperidol) has been more extensively studied. Serious adverse effects associated with neuroleptic treatment include restlessness (**akathisia**), **parkinsonism,** acute dystonias, and **neuroleptic malignant syndrome (NMS).** The most detrimental consequence of long-term neuroleptic use is the development of involuntary motor movements (**TK**). Other adverse effects include **anticholinergic effects, orthostatic hypotension, sedation,** and **hyperprolactinemia.** The gold standard for treatment-refractory schizophrenia is **clozapine;** however, its use is limited due to a **1% to 2% risk of agranulocytosis** and consequent need for frequent blood monitoring. Atypical neuroleptics are associated with lower rates of extrapyramidal effects but have the potential to produce "metabolic syndrome" associated with impaired glucose regulation and obesity.

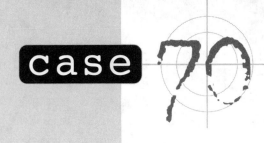

case 70

CC   A 25-year-old woman with a **history of depression** is brought to the ER by her boyfriend after she attempted to run into traffic.

HPI   Her boyfriend notes that she suffers from depressive episodes occurring about twice per year, each lasting for about 2 months. During these periods of depression she talks about **odd beliefs,** writes in her journal, mumbles to herself, and **seems disorganized.** Her most recent depression resolved about 6 weeks ago. She has no history of manic symptoms.

During the past 3 weeks, the patient has become increasingly convinced that she is pregnant, although she has not been sexually active. Despite multiple negative pregnancy tests and a reassuring visit to her gynecologist, she **continues to believe she is pregnant.** Her boyfriend notes that she has been writing in her journal lately, but her writing is **disorganized and illegible.** Earlier today, while waiting for the bus, she began mumbling to herself before suddenly running into traffic, although she was not harmed.

PE   Physical exam normal. On mental status exam, she seems calm but **guarded,** avoiding sustained eye contact. She endorses **auditory hallucinations** (reporting that they had told her to run into traffic) and continues to insist that she is pregnant "with the divine child." She denies thoughts of self-harm or of harming others. She describes her mood as "fine."

Labs Urine and serum toxicology screens negative. HCG: negative.

case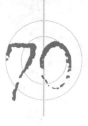

Schizoaffective Disorder

Differential | Major depressive disorder with psychotic features or **bipolar disorder with psychotic features** may be difficult to differentiate from schizoaffective disorder. The key diagnostic factor is that **schizoaffective disorder features psychotic symptoms in the absence of mood symptoms.** In both major depressive disorder and bipolar disorder with psychotic features, psychotic symptoms occur only in the setting of mood symptoms.

Pathogenesis | Schizoaffective disorder prominently features **both affective and psychotic symptoms.** For diagnosis, criteria for either a major depressive or manic episode must be met, and the patient must have also experienced **delusions or hallucinations in the absence of the mood symptoms.**

Epidemiology | The prevalence of schizoaffective disorder is less than 1%, and it affects women more often than men. Prognosis is better than that of schizophrenia.

Management | Patients with schizoaffective disorder can benefit from psychotherapy and pharmacologic treatment. Neuroleptics can be used to target symptoms of psychosis and stabilize mood. Depending on the subtype (bipolar versus depressed), patients might also benefit from a mood stabilizer or antidepressant.

Breakout Point

> **Pseudocyesis** is the name given to a delusion of pregnancy accompanied by physiologic changes congruent with actual pregnancy. **Couvade syndrome** describes symptoms of pregnancy in husbands of pregnant women.

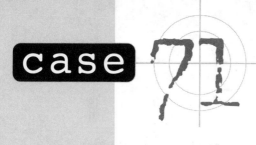

CC A 24-year-old man presents to a local plastic surgeon for corrective surgery of his "ugly nose."

HPI He states he is frustrated and anxious due to his perceived defect. He stays at home to **avoid other people** because he fears they will stare at him. He also reports spending several hours a day **examining his nose** in the mirror and applying makeup to make his nose "less noticeable." His past medical history is significant for **three rhinoplasties.**

PE Nose appears symmetrical without gross abnormality.

case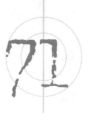

Body Dysmorphic Disorder (BDD)

Differential

Delusional disorder, somatic type is diagnosed when the belief is rigid, unshakable, and held with **delusional intensity**.

Anorexia nervosa or **bulimia nervosa** should be considered when concerns center on body weight and the patient engages in behaviors intended to reduce weight.

Gender identity disorder is marked by bodily discomfort due to a desire to be the other sex.

OCD is not diagnosed when the only symptom is preoccupation with appearance.

Mood and anxiety disorders have high comorbidity with BDD. Care should be taken to screen for symptoms of depression and anxiety.

Pathogenesis

BDD involves an **intense preoccupation with an imagined defect in appearance** that causes significant distress or marked social/occupational impairment. The etiology of BDD is unknown, but high comorbidity with mood disorders and OCDs is suggestive of serotonergic pathology.

Epidemiology

Prevalence is uncertain, but BDD has been estimated to account for 2% of visits to plastic surgeons. **Women are affected more often** than men, with an age of onset typically between 15 and 30 years.

Management

SSRIs or other serotonergic agents (clomipramine) may be the **most effective** pharmacologic approach. **Neuroleptics** (pimozide) may also be used. **Psychotherapy** (eg, CBT addressing unwanted thoughts and behaviors, or psychodynamic therapy examining the dynamic basis of symptoms) is also indicated.

Breakout Point

Most Common Foci of Imagined Defects in BDD
Hair
Nose
Skin
Eyes

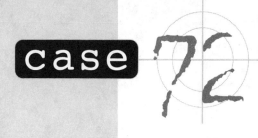

case 72

CC   A 17-year-old **woman** is brought to the ER with paralysis of her lower extremities.

HPI   The patient is accompanied by her mother, who reports that her daughter **witnessed the shooting of her boyfriend** yesterday. The patient's mother says that the motor weakness started after the incident and has progressed to total paralysis below the waist, although she reports normal bladder and bowel function. Oddly, she seems **unconcerned with her symptoms.**

PE   Normal muscle tone in all extremities; 2+ reflexes throughout; no flaccidity or fasciculations; sensory function intact throughout.

Labs   Normal.

Imaging   MR imaging, lumbar spine: normal.

case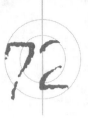

Conversion Disorder

Differential

Neurologic illness must be ruled out with appropriate medical workup.

Somatization disorder requires the presence of four pain symptoms, two GI symptoms, one sexual symptom, and one pseudoneurologic symptom unrelated to a medical condition.

Pain disorder involves only symptoms of pain with no apparent cause or pain in excess of known organic pathology.

Pathogenesis

Conversion disorder presents with sensory or motor complaints suggestive of neurological illness (usually **paralysis, blindness,** or **mutism**) that are **unintentionally produced,** cannot be explained by an organic etiology, and are usually **associated with a psychological precipitant.** This patient may have been so afraid during the shooting that she wanted to run away, abandoning her boyfriend, which created a psychological conflict resolved by loss of strength in her legs. **La belle indifférence** describes the classic finding of the patients' inappropriately low level of concern for their condition.

Epidemiology

Conversion disorder is associated with **female gender,** lower socioeconomic status, and **lower levels of education.**

Management

Symptoms should be allowed to resolve without invoking shame; **patients should not be told that their symptoms are all in the mind.** Inform patients that their symptoms are very real despite the lack of organic evidence to explain them. Patients should be reassured that the prognosis is good, function should gradually return, and permanent loss of function is rare. Symptoms typically last up to a week and remit spontaneously. In refractory cases, amobarbital ("truth serum") or lorazepam can be used to help engage the patient in therapy.

Breakout Point

> Pseudoseizures, also known as nonelectrical seizures, are a manifestation of conversion disorder that typically approximate a generalized tonic-clonic seizure. The nonelectrical etiology of the event may be evident from history or exam, but more sophisticated cases may require long-term EEG monitoring in order to obtain an EEG recording during the event.

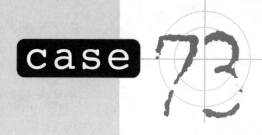

case 73

CC A 26-year-old male nurse's aide presents to a gastroen-terologist concerned that he has hepatitis. He reports that he drank water from a garden hose approximately **6 months** ago and has since experienced abdominal discomfort. Although he has received **appropriate medical evaluation** from his primary care physician, with **reassurance that he has no medical illness**, his preoccupation has continued.

HPI The patient denies any anorexia, diarrhea, or malaise. Additionally, he has no risk factors for hepatitis. Despite numerous benign medical workups and unremarkable laboratory values, he **continues to fear** that he has undetected hepatitis. He reports abdominal discomfort and gas after eating large meals, which he attributes to a flourishing hepatitis infection that is "destroying" his liver.

PE Physical and neurologic exams normal.

Labs Lytes/CBC: normal. TFTs: normal; anti-HAV (IgG and IgM) negative; HBcAg negative; HBsAg negative; no heterophil antibodies.

case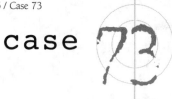

Hypochondriasis

Differential

General medical conditions may present with nonspecific symptoms; therefore, a thorough medical evaluation to rule out serious pathology is warranted in every case.

Somatization disorder requires the presence of four pain symptoms, two GI symptoms, one sexual symptom, and one pseudoneurologic symptom unrelated to a medical condition.

Delusional disorder, somatic type is focused on a specific somatic perception, whereas hypochondriasis features a fear of having a medical illness.

Other major psychiatric disorders may require distinguishing affective and anxiety disorders with somatic preoccupations from hypochondriasis.

Pathogenesis

Hypochondriasis involves a persistent **preoccupation with (or fear of) medical illness,** despite appropriate medical evaluation and reassurance, **lasting for at least 6 months.** Current understanding of the etiology of hypochondriasis emphasizes poor tolerance and **amplification of normal bodily sensations.**

Epidemiology

Prevalence in general medical clinics has been estimated to be as high as 5% to 10%, with males and females equally affected. Age at onset is usually between 20 and 30 years.

Management

Patients should undergo thorough assessment for comorbid psychiatric and medical illnesses. Once medical illness has been ruled out, **frequent regularly scheduled appointments** with their physician may help ease anxiety and limit the need for unscheduled visits. Invasive diagnostic or therapeutic procedures should be limited. Patients with hypochondriasis are usually resistant to psychiatric referral, but aggressive treatment of any underlying depressive and anxious symptoms may decrease complaints.

Breakout Point

> Three percent of medical students experience symptoms of hypochondriasis, usually during the first 2 years of medical school.

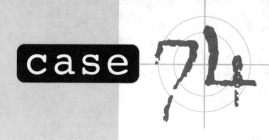

case

CC A **25-year-old woman** presents to a new internist complaining that her previous physician "didn't take me seriously."

HPI She has made **multiple visits** and phone calls to her primary care physician over the past few years, undergoing extensive evaluations for a variety of **painful complaints**, including **headaches, menstrual cramps, joint pains,** and **chest pain.** In addition, she has seen various specialists for **nausea and diarrhea, impaired sexual arousal,** and **double vision,** without any objective evidence of medical illness.

PE Normal.

Labs Lytes/CBC: normal. TFTs: normal; RPR/VDRL nonreactive; β-hCG negative for pregnancy; ESR: normal; rheumatoid factor and ANA negative.

case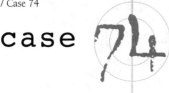

Somatization Disorder

Differential

General medical conditions may mean that a thorough medical workup is indicated to rule out possible medical etiologies.

Undifferentiated somatoform disorder applies to patients with one or more somatic complaints but fewer than the eight required for somatization disorder.

Conversion disorder involves one or more symptoms of neurologic origin that are associated with psychological stressors.

Hypochondriasis features prominent fear that one has a serious medical illness based on a misinterpretation of physical symptoms.

Factitious disorder and malingering involve symptoms that are intentionally feigned for secondary gain (malingering) or for assumption of sick role as a primary motivation (factitious disorder).

Pathogenesis

Somatization disorder involves a history of multiple physical complaints not attributed to medical illness **beginning before age 30 years**, including at least **four pain symptoms, two GI symptoms, one sexual symptom,** and **one pseudoneurologic symptom** (excluding pain), which are **not deliberately or consciously produced.** Etiology is unknown, but numerous biological and psychological theories have been proposed. Comorbidity with other psychiatric disorders is common. Numerous unnecessary invasive procedures are often performed before this disorder is recognized.

Epidemiology

Lifetime prevalence is 0.5%, with **females affected more than males by 5:1.**

Management

Once medical illness has been ruled out, **frequent regularly scheduled appointments** with a physician may help ease anxiety and limit the need for unscheduled visits. The patient should be reassured that their complaints, although valid, are not the result of a serious medical condition. **Psychotherapy** has been shown to decrease health care costs by 50%. Pharmacotherapy should target symptoms of any comorbid psychiatric disorders.

Breakout Point

Diagnostic Criteria for Somatization Disorder (Prays 4 Good 2 Superb Nursing)
Pain Symptoms – 4 **G**astrointestinal Symptoms – 2 **S**exual Symptom – 1 **N**eurological Symptom – 1

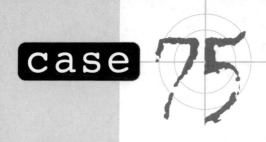

case

CC A 35-year-old woman presents to a psychiatrist's office with feelings of "guilt and anxiety." As the interview is drawing to a close, she blurts out that she was **arrested for shoplifting 1 week ago.**

HPI The patient recounts a history of **recurrent, impulsive stealing** since she was 16 years of age. She had never been arrested until she was recently caught at a local department store putting several key chains in her purse. She states that she **had no need for these items** and certainly could afford them because she has a well-paying job working as an attorney. She states that the frequency of her stealing has waxed and waned over the years. She emphasizes that she has a **sense of building tension** before committing the theft, which is **only relieved once she has stolen something.** Guilt then follows each episode, and she quickly drives to a local charity's thrift store and donates the items.

case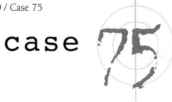

Kleptomania

Differential

Impulsive or injudicious behavior, such as shoplifting, can be a symptom of **mania, psychosis, substance abuse, or personality disorders** (especially antisocial personality disorder). Although a diagnosis of kleptomania requires that stealing is not a result of another diagnosis, patients with kleptomania may nonetheless have other comorbid psychiatric diagnoses.

Pathogenesis

Kleptomania is categorized in the DSM-IV as an impulse-control disorder not classified elsewhere. Essential features include **recurrent stealing of items** that a person **does not need, escalating tension** immediately before the theft, and a **sense of pleasure or relief** at the time of the theft. The DSM-IV is also careful to note that the theft **is not committed as an act of anger or vengeance and is not due to a delusion or hallucination.**

Epidemiology

The exact prevalence is unknown, but kleptomania is thought to account for only a small percent of all shoplifters.

Management

Kleptomania is rare, so large studies of treatment have not been performed. **Psychotherapy** may range from insight-oriented to CBTs. Pharmacological treatment may involve **SSRIs, TCAs,** or **mood stabilizers.**

Breakout Point

> When caught, male patients with kleptomania are more likely to be imprisoned, whereas female patients are more likely to be referred for psychiatric evaluation.

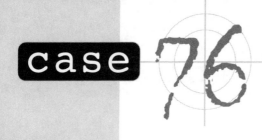

case 76

CC A 19-year-old college student presents to the campus health clinic with a complaint of "hair loss."

HPI When asked about her hair loss, the patient appears embarrassed and tearful explaining that she "pulls it out," describing it as a "habit I just can't kick." She states that when she is studying or watching TV she has an **"urge to pluck" her hair,** and she finds it **"hard to resist the temptation,"** especially when she is alone. She describes **spending excessive amounts of time concealing her hair loss** "so no one finds out." She endorses feeling ashamed of her behavior, stating "I know I shouldn't do it, but it **feels good in the moment."**

PE Physical exam reveals a young woman with heavy eye makeup **concealing sparse eyebrow hairs and only a few short eyelashes on the eyelids.** Exam of the scalp reveals patchy areas of hair loss featuring a **combination of long, normal hairs and short, broken strands.**

case

Trichotillomania

Differential

Medical causes of hair loss should be considered, including dermatologic, infectious, and endocrine disorders.

OCD may present with compulsions to pull or pluck hair, although this is usually associated with some obsessive thought and is not typically associated with any pleasure or gratification.

Pathogenesis

Trichotillomania is classified in the DSM-IV as an "impulse control disorder not elsewhere classified." The criteria include **noticeable hair loss due to plucking/pulling**, an **associated tension before pulling out or when trying to resist** pulling, **pleasure or gratification** associated with pulling, and **interference with daily functioning**. The course of trichotillomania varies, may wax and wane, and could last for years. Hair pulling may occur with **any area of the body** but most is most often associated with the **eyelashes, eyebrows, and scalp.**

Management

Many different pharmacologic and psychotherapeutic techniques are employed in the treatment of trichotillomania with variable success. **SSRIs** are commonly used, but many classes of medications including benzodiazepines and neuroleptics **(pimozide)** have also been employed. Other interventions that have been helpful are **hypnosis and behavioral therapy,** including **biofeedback** (monitoring of physiological functions in order to learn better control of them).

Breakout Point

> Other impulse control disorders described by the DSM-IV include intermittent explosive disorder, kleptomania, pyromania, and (by far the most common) pathological gambling.

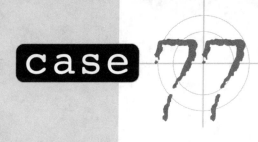

case 77

CC A 34-year-old man presenting for his annual physical exam admits that his **6-year marriage** is somewhat troubled, stating, "things just aren't what they used to be in the bedroom."

HPI On further questioning, he reveals that he is interested in sex only when **wearing his wife's panties and negligees.** "I don't know what's wrong with me." He reports that his wife is quite upset by this behavior, and they have not had sex in more than 6 months. Now he needs to be dressed in his wife's clothing to reach orgasm while masturbating. He denies any symptoms that are consistent with depression, anxiety, or psychosis. His childhood was unremarkable, and he no past history of psychiatric illness. He has **no history of homosexual relationships.**

case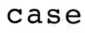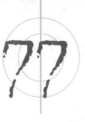

Transvestic Fetishism

Differential

Gender identity disorder involves a strong and persistent cross-gender identification and a desire to be the other sex. Cross-dressing may feature in gender identity disorder, but it is not associated with sexual arousal as it is in transvestic fetishism.

Homosexuality is considered a normal variant of accepted sexual behavior and is not typically associated with transvestic fetishism.

Pathogenesis

Paraphilias are abnormal expressions of sexuality that feature **at least 6 months** of unusual, recurrent, intense sexual fantasies, urges, or behaviors. The etiology of paraphilia is unknown. **Transvestic fetishism** is a paraphilia that involves a heterosexual male cross-dressing in women's clothes. Articles of clothing are used in masturbation and in intercourse. The cross-dressing may minimize anxiety associated with sexual intimacy. When not dressed in women's clothes, the male is usually unremarkably masculine. Some individuals with transvestic fetishism also have gender dysphoria.

Management

Individual psychotherapy (to address any underlying reasons for this behavior) and **couple's counseling** (to address marital problems that this behavior may be causing) are both indicated.

Breakout Point

Paraphilias Categorized under Paraphilia not Otherwise Specified in the DSM-IV
Telephone Scatologia: Obscene Phone Calls
Necrophilia: Corpses
Partialism: Extreme Focus on One Part of the Body (eg, feet)
Zoophilia: Animals
Coprophilia: Feces
Klismaphilia: Enemas
Urophilia: Urine

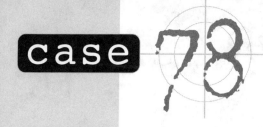

case 78

CC   A 19-year-old man presents to the ER after being punched in the eye by a stranger on the subway.

HPI   When questioned about the incident he initially denies any precipitant to the attack but finally admits that he had **"gotten too close"** to a woman (whom he had never met). When pressed to explain, he reports that he **touched the woman's breasts** and **rubbed his genitals against her thighs.** He reported sheepishly that "I always do this stuff when I'm **on the subway**— it's so crowded and usually nobody notices." The patient is a predentistry college student with a 3.8 grade point average and **no criminal history.** He has never been in a serious relationship. He denies any symptoms consistent with depression, mania, anxiety, or psychosis.

PE   Notable for erythema and swelling around the right eye.

case 78

Frotteurism

Differential

Mania is often associated with hypersexuality but also features elevated mood, pressured speech, racing thoughts, and grandiosity.

Substance intoxication resulting from many drugs, such as alcohol, amphetamines, ketamine, and MDMA (ecstasy), can lead to hypersexuality and inappropriate behaviors.

Brain injury, particularly of the frontal lobes, can result in disinhibition, hypersexuality, and inappropriate behavior.

Pathogenesis

Paraphilias are abnormal expressions of sexuality that feature **at least 6 months** of unusual, recurrent, intense sexual fantasies, urges, or behaviors. The etiology of paraphilia is unknown. **Frotteurism** is a paraphilia which involves **touching and rubbing against a nonconsenting individual.** Such behavior most commonly occurs in crowded places where the person can more easily escape detection. Often, the person engaging in frottage fantasizes about having a relationship with this person. Frotteurism often begins by adolescence, and most acts occur between the ages of 15 and 25 years.

Management

CBT directed toward the extinction of these behaviors are the mainstay of treatment. **High-dose SSRIs** may be used to diminish libido. In extreme cases, depot medroxyprogesterone (Depo-Provera) can be used to decrease libido.

Breakout Point

Paraphilias Specified by the DSM-IV

Exhibitionism: Exposing Genitalia to an Unsuspecting Stranger

Fetishism: Focus on, or Use of, Nonliving Objects

Frotteurism: Touching or Rubbing against a Nonconsenting Person

Pedophilia: Sexual Activity with a Prepubescent Child

Sexual Masochism: Acts of Being Humiliated, Beaten, Bound, or Otherwise Made to Suffer

Sexual Sadism: Acts in Which Psychological or Physical Suffering of Another Person Is Sexually Exciting

Transvestic Fetishism: Cross-Dressing in a Heterosexual Male

Voyeurism: Observing an Unsuspecting Person Who Is Naked, Disrobing, or Engaging in Sexual Activity

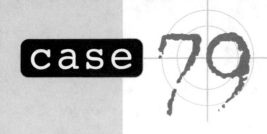

case 79

CC A 34-year-old woman presents to her primary care physician with tearfulness, abdominal pain, and chronic depressed mood.

HPI She finds herself "worrying all the time" and "having trouble focusing at work." She reports **feeling "worthless,"** and that she **"can't do anything right."** She states that "things are tense" with her boyfriend, and she **"feels isolated"** from her friends and family members. Becoming concerned, her primary care provider states **"I'm worried someone is hurting you."** The patient then reports that 6 months ago **her boyfriend started demeaning her in public, criticizing** her hair and dress. Soon he started **limiting her contact** with close friends and about 1 month ago he began **grabbing, slapping, and pushing** her in anger. He would follow the abuse with profuse apologies. The patient concludes with "I can't believe this, he was so nice in the beginning."

PE Exam reveals a tearful woman with a bruise on her upper arm.

ABUSE

case 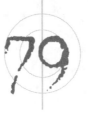 79

Domestic Violence

Differential

Victims of domestic violence **may come to medical attention** during hospital visits for sexual trauma, somatic complaints, or strange injuries that the victim cannot explain. **Patients may present initially with psychiatric complaints** of depression, dissociation, anxiety, substance abuse, adjustment disorders, suicidality, or homicidality.

Pathogenesis

Domestic violence occurs when an intimate partner of the **same or opposite sex** exerts **power or control over the victim by physical or sexual violence, coercion, isolation, control, or threats.** There are no specific predictors for who will become a victim of domestic violence. Perpetrators, however, often have a history of exposure to violence in their own families and have been violent in prior relationships.

Management

Routine screening by health care providers (either **verbal or written**) should be conducted in a **private space.** The questions may be general screening questions, or more direct questions if abuse is suspected. **Confidentiality and entries in the medical record** should be discussed. **Questioning should be nonjudgmental.** The treating clinician should be able to help with safety planning and information about the local resources for local domestic violence shelters and treatment. The clinician should appreciate the **risks facing the victim who is considering leaving** the batterer and the **victim's wishes regarding this decision should be respected.**

Breakout Point

> Asking the questions **"Do you ever feel unsafe at home?"** and **"Has anyone at home hit you or tried to injure you in any way?"** has a sensitivity of 71% and a specificity of 85% in detecting domestic violence.

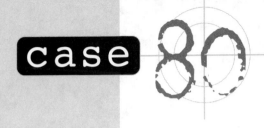

case 80

CC An 82-year-old man is brought to the ER by his son who notes that his father fell at home.

HPI The patient has diagnoses of Alzheimer dementia, hypertension, and IDDM, and he is not able to provide a coherent history. He cries throughout the exam, repeating the phrase "**help me.**" His son is reluctant to speak with ER staff, simply stating "that bastard did it again—I give him a home, I do everything for him, and he keeps on falling and ruining my life." His son is **unable to provide specific details** about the fall. With continued questioning, the son becomes increasingly agitated, stating, "Just fix him up so we can go." The ER nurse notes the smell alcohol on the son's breath. Hospital records reveal that the patient has been in the ER several times this year—three times for poorly substantiated falls and two times for significant hyperglycemia.

PE VS: no fever; hypertension (to 162/101); tachycardia (to 111). The patient is disheveled and malodorous, wearing soiled, wet clothes. His left upper arm is bruised, and his left forearm has several healed bruises.

Labs Hct: 34, platelets, 125; sodium, 147; BUN, 41; creatinine, 1.2; glucose, 352.

Imaging XRs: notable for **fractured left humerus**, newly healed **fractured right ulna, and healing right metacarpals.** CT, head: **small frontal subdural hematoma.**

ABUSE

case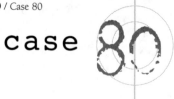

Elder Abuse

Differential

Dementia may progress to the point that, despite well-intentioned care by family, the patient is no longer safe to live at home because of impulsive behaviors and risk of falls. Even the most vigilant family members find it extremely difficult to provide the 24-hour care these patients require.

Medical causes of falls, including orthostatic hypotension and peripheral neuropathy, should be investigated.

Pathogenesis

Under any circumstances, caring for a medically ill, dependent elderly individual can be extremely stressful for a caregiver. Such difficult situations may be exacerbated by feelings of frustration and despair, as well as ambivalence about the relationship with the patient. Caregivers may become abusive or neglectful, particularly in the context of a lack of support and loss of control over the situation. Abusive caregivers have often been abused themselves.

Management

In cases of elder abuse, the priority is to provide appropriate medical treatment and ensure the safety of the patient. Many states have **mandated reporting of elder abuse** to the appropriate authority. Appropriate care usually involves interdisciplinary cooperation between the medical team, social services, and state agencies.

Breakout Point

Warning Signs of Elder Abuse
• Unexplained Falls, Burns, Fractures
• Bruises in Unusual Areas
• Inappropriate Administration of Medication by Caregiver
• Disparity between Family Financial Assets and Patient's Living Condition
• Excessive Caregiver Stress
• History of Family Violence

questions

1. A 27-year-old man with uncertain psychiatric history is brought to the ER after his roommate calls for an ambulance, concerned that he has "overdosed on all his pills." The patient is grossly confused and is unable to report what he might have ingested. On exam, he is febrile to 40°C, hypertensive to 200/110, and tachycardic to 120, and he has marked rigidity of his limbs. The medication most likely to be responsible for his presentation is

   A. Lithium
   B. Fluoxetine
   C. Risperidone
   D. Buspirone
   E. Chlordiazepoxide

2. A 45-year-old woman with no prior psychiatric history presents to her primary care physician requesting surgery "to remove the parasites from my belly." She reports that she has felt "something moving" in her abdomen for the past 2 months, and believes that she is "infested by worms." Despite her sense of discomfort, she notes that she has been able to continue her work as an elementary school-teacher. β-HCG is negative; complete physical examination and abdominal US are unrevealing. The most appropriate diagnosis is

   A. Hypochondriasis
   B. Somatization disorder
   C. Brief psychotic disorder
   D. Schizophrenia
   E. Delusional disorder

3. A 32-year-old man with a history of bipolar I disorder is brought to the ER with blurred vision, tremor, and confusion. A lithium level is returned at an elevated level of 3.4. Treatment should include

   A. Cyproheptadine
   B. Hemodialysis
   C. Dantrolene
   D. Cooling blankets
   E. Activated charcoal

4. A 17-year-old man is brought to the ER after being found unresponsive in the bathroom at school. He is sluggishly responsive to noxious stimuli, and physical exam reveals perioral cyanosis and pinpoint pupils. The appropriate medication to administer is

   A. Buprenorphine
   B. Naloxone
   C. Methadone
   D. Naltrexone
   E. Levo-α-acetylmethadol

5. A 52-year-old man with no prior psychiatric history is referred to the psychiatry clinic by his primary care physician who is concerned with his worsening paranoia and auditory hallucinations. Since losing his job 1 year ago, the patient has taken no pleasure in his usual activities and has suffered insomnia, poor appetite (with a 20 lb-weight loss), fatigue, and feelings of guilt over not being able to provide for his family. More recently, he has reported hearing unfamiliar voices discussing his situation and calling him "worthless." He voices a belief that he was fired from his job because governmental agencies are conspiring against him. The most appropriate diagnosis is

   A. Adjustment disorder with depressed mood
   B. Schizophreniform disorder
   C. Schizoaffective disorder, depressive type
   D. Major depressive disorder with psychotic features
   E. Bipolar I disorder

6. A 41-year-old man is brought to the ER by police for treatment of lacerations to his forearm. The patient had been arrested a few days earlier and had been remanded to jail to await trial. This afternoon, he used a pen to cut his left forearm three times. The lacerations are sufficiently deep to require sutures. On exam, the patient freely admits causing the injury himself. He denies depressed mood or any symptoms of psychosis. As the ER staff attend to his injuries, the patient is noted to be happily feeding himself from his dinner tray, reading a magazine given to him by nursing staff. The most appropriate diagnosis is

   A. Malingering
   B. Factitious disorder
   C. Borderline personality disorder
   D. Sexual masochism
   E. Trichotillomania

7. A 28-year-old woman with a history of depression is brought to the ER complaining of a throbbing headache and is found to be acutely hypertensive to 210/105, tachycardic to 120, and confused. Her boyfriend reports that her symptoms began shortly after they dined at an Italian restaurant. The medication most likely to be responsible for her symptoms is

   A. Fluoxetine
   B. Bupropion
   C. Buspirone
   D. Tranylcypromine
   E. Nortriptyline

8. A 17-year-old high school senior is admitted to the hospital due to chronic weight loss over the past year, now resulting in her weighing 73% of her ideal body weight. She appears cachectic, but she endorses a belief that she is "disgustingly fat" and reports that she had been restricting her caloric intake. With the permission of her parents, tube feedings are initiated at 2400 kcal/day in an attempt to help her gain weight. On the third hospital day, the patient is noted to be lethargic, confused, and tachycardic. These symptoms are most closely related to abnormalities in which of the following laboratory values

   A. Sodium and bicarbonate
   B. Potassium and chloride
   C. Magnesium and phosphate
   D. Calcium and chloride
   E. BUN and creatinine

9. A 72-year-old man with mild Alzheimer dementia is admitted to the hospital with symptoms of bloody stool, fatigue, and a 30 lb-weight loss over the preceding 3 months. On colonoscopy, he is found to have advanced adenocarcinoma of the colon. When this finding is discussed with him, he refuses any surgical intervention, noting that he understands he has cancer, and surgery may prolong his life, but "I don't want to spend the rest of my time sitting in the hospital. I know you want to help me, but I just want to go home and die in peace." He maintains this opinion over several days, despite the objections of his daughter, who is his health care proxy. Psychiatric examination reveals mild deficits in short-term memory and visuospatial functioning, appropriate sadness, but no evidence of depression. The appropriate course of action would be to

A. Honor the patient's wishes and allow him to go home
B. Defer the decision to the daughter due to the diagnosis of Alzheimer dementia
C. Proceed with surgery on the basis of the ethical principle of beneficence
D. Keep the patient in the hospital for another week to see if he changes his mind
E. Ask the hospital attorney to file for a court-appointed guardian for the patient

10. A 28-year-old woman undergoing evaluation for a work-related injury signs a release requesting that her physician fax her records to her attorney. After faxing the documents, the physician realizes that she has faxed them to the wrong number. The physician's chief responsibility is to

A. Document the error in the chart
B. Inform the patient of the error
C. Ascertain the destination of the erroneous fax
D. Institute a more reliable system of transmitting medical information
E. Request another signed release from the patient

11. A 22-year-old man is brought to the ER by his roommates who are concerned that for the past 10 days he has been talking rapidly, not sleeping, and spending large amounts of money buying computer components on the Internet for a "machine that will solve the world's problems." First-line pharmacotherapy for this patient would include

A. Fluoxetine
B. Phenelzine
C. Nortriptyline
D. Bupropion
E. Lithium

12. A 19-year-old female college student presents to the student health clinic, at the prompting of her boyfriend, with a complaint of extreme anxiety about her classes. She notes that she is doing very well with her assignments outside of class but is worried that she is going to fail two of her courses because they each require an oral presentation in front of the class. She states that she will not be able to do this because "everyone will think that I'm stupid," although she recognizes that "it doesn't make any sense." The most likely diagnosis is

A. GAD
B. Avoidant personality disorder
C. Social phobia
D. Panic disorder with agoraphobia
E. Specific phobia

13. A 33-year-old woman presents to the ER with multiple injuries that she reports are due to falling down a flight of stairs at home. The pattern of injuries, which include a fractured left radius, bruised right thigh, and broken nose, do not seem congruent with her story. When directly asked about domestic violence, she admits being beaten by her husband. The appropriate course of action is to

A. Call the police to arrest the husband
B. Refer the patient and her husband to couple's therapy
C. Tell the patient that spousal abuse is grounds for divorce and she should leave her husband
D. Educate the patient about domestic violence and the options available to maintain her safety
E. Provide psychiatric hospitalization to the patient for her own protection

14. A 27-year-old man presents to the psychiatry clinic concerned that he is only able to reach orgasm if he is holding a pair of his wife's high-heeled shoes. The patient denies any interest in wearing the shoes, but notes that he finds touching and rubbing them arousing. The most appropriate diagnosis is

A. Fetishism
B. Transvestic fetishism
C. Frotteurism
D. Exhibitionism
E. Paraphilia not otherwise specified

15. A 44-year-old man with schizophrenia, paranoid type, is found to have a WBC of 2.9 with 40% neutrophils on routing blood testing. The medication most likely responsible for this finding is

A. Olanzapine
B. Clozapine
C. Quetiapine
D. Aripiprazole
E. Risperidone

16. A 39-year-old woman with schizoaffective disorder, recently started on risperidone, presents for a scheduled appointment with her psychiatrist appearing restless, uncomfortable, and unable to stay seated for more than a minute at a time. She reports a sense of "not being able to stop moving." The appropriate treatment is

A. Benztropine
B. Diphenhydramine
C. Increased risperidone
D. Haloperidol
E. Propranolol

17. A 72-year-old woman is admitted for surgical repair of a fractured hip. On the second postoperative day, she is noted to be confused and agitated, and olanzapine is started. A subsequent ECG reveals a QTc of 510 ms. Which of the following values should be closely monitored in this setting?

    A. Potassium and magnesium
    B. Sodium and calcium
    C. Phosphate and bicarbonate
    D. BUN and creatinine
    E. Glucose and chloride

18. A 21-year-old man is brought to the ER by police after they were called by his neighbors who were concerned after they heard loud crashing coming from his apartment. When they arrived, they report that the patient was extremely agitated, throwing furniture, and required multiple officers to restrain him. His urine toxicology screen is positive for PCP. Which receptor does PCP primarily act on?

    A. GABA
    B. Acetylcholine
    C. NMDA
    D. Norepinephrine
    E. Serotonin

19. A 16-year-old boy is referred for psychiatric evaluation due to frequent fighting at school. He has a long history of disciplinary problems, including stealing money from other students, truancy, and vandalism. The most appropriate diagnosis is

    A. ADHD
    B. Oppositional defiant disorder
    C. Antisocial personality disorder
    D. Narcissistic personality disorder
    E. Conduct disorder

20. A 45-year-old man is admitted with cholecystitis. On the third hospital day he is noted to be anxious, confused, tremulous, and diaphoretic. On PE, he is tachycardic to 120 and hypertensive to 180/90. His LFTs are elevated with a 2:1 ratio of AST to ALT, and his CBC reveals a macrocytic anemia. Urgent treatment should include

    A. Disulfiram
    B. Citalopram
    C. Naltrexone
    D. Acamprosate
    E. Chlordiazepoxide

answers

1-C

A. Lithium [incorrect]. The patient is presenting with symptoms of neuroleptic malignant syndrome (NMS), and lithium is not a neuroleptic.

B. Fluoxetine [incorrect]. This patient is presenting with symptoms of NMS. Fluoxetine is not a neuroleptic and therefore would not be responsible for this presentation.

C. Risperidone [correct]. The patient is presenting with delirium, fever, rigidity, and autonomic instability—all symptoms of NMS. Laboratory testing would be likely to reveal leukocytosis and elevation of CPK. NMS occurs in response to dopamine antagonism, usually in the setting of increased neuroleptic use or overdose. Of the agents listed, risperidone is the only neuroleptic.

D. Buspirone [incorrect]. This patient is presenting with symptoms of NMS. Buspirone is not a neuroleptic and therefore would not be responsible for this presentation.

E. Chlordiazepoxide [incorrect]. This patient is presenting with symptoms of NMS. Chlordiazepoxide is not a neuroleptic and therefore would not be responsible for this presentation.

2-E

A. Hypochondriasis [incorrect]. This condition is characterized by a recurrent fear of medical illness, occurring over at least 6 months, despite medical reassurance of health. Hypochondriasis tends to be more focused on the general idea of being medically ill rather on one particular physical symptom.

B. Somatization disorder [incorrect]. This diagnosis requires a constellation of unexplained symptoms, including at least four pain symptoms, two GI symptoms, one sexual symptom, and one pseudoneurological symptom.

C. Brief psychotic disorder [incorrect]. This condition is diagnosed when psychotic symptoms occur for at least 1 day, but not more than 1 month.

D. Schizophrenia [incorrect]. This condition requires the presence of at least two symptoms of psychosis over a period greater than 1 month that cause marked impairment in functioning.

E. Delusional disorder [correct]. At least one month of nonbizarre (ie, could realistically occur) delusional beliefs, in the absence of other symptoms of psychosis or marked impact on daily functioning, is most congruent with a diagnosis of delusional disorder (in this case, somatic type).

3-B

A. Cyproheptadine [incorrect]. This is not indicated for treatment of lithium toxicity.

B. Hemodialysis [correct]. Lithium toxicity at levels greater than 2.5 requires hemodialysis. At lithium levels below 2.5, treatment decisions are based on severity of clinical symptoms. None of the other agents listed is indicated for treatment of lithium toxicity.

C. Dantrolene [incorrect]. This is not indicated for treatment of lithium toxicity.

D. Cooling blankets [incorrect]. These are not indicated for treatment of lithium toxicity.

E. Activated charcoal [incorrect]. This is not indicated for treatment of lithium toxicity.

4-B

A. Buprenorphine [incorrect]. This is a partial agonist at the opioid receptor that can be used for treatment of opiate withdrawal or long-term maintenance treatment.

B. Naloxone [correct]. The patient is presenting with the signs and symptoms of opiate toxicity, likely due to overdose. Naloxone is an opiate antagonist that can be administered intravenously to reverse the respiratory depression and other effects of opiate toxicity.

C. Methadone [incorrect] is a long-acting opiate agonist frequently used for treatment of opiate withdrawal or long-term maintenance treatment.

D. Naltrexone [incorrect]. This is an opioid antagonist available in oral formulation that is used in long-term treatment of substance dependence.

E. Levo-α-acetylmethadol [incorrect]. This is a rarely used ultra-long-acting opiate agonist.

5-D

A. Adjustment disorder with depressed mood [incorrect]. The diagnostic criteria for adjustment disorder require that the symptoms do not meet criteria for another disorder. In this case, the symptoms meet the criteria for major depressive disorder.

B. Schizophreniform disorder [incorrect]. This diagnosis describes symptoms of schizophrenia occurring for more than 1 month but less than the 6 months required for a diagnosis of schizophrenia. The DSM-IV specifies that psychotic symptoms related to a mood episode do not meet diagnostic criteria.

C. Schizoaffective disorder, depressive type [incorrect]. Like schizophreniform disorder, this condition includes both affective and psychotic symptoms; however, diagnosis requires the occurrence of psychotic symptoms for a period of at least 2 weeks in the absence of any mood symptoms.

D. Major depressive disorder with psychotic features [correct]. The patient has experienced five or more of the symptoms of depression (specifically anhedonia, disturbance of sleep, decrease in appetite, fatigue, and guilt) for a period greater than 2 weeks. His development of psychotic symptoms (paranoia and hallucinations) has occurred solely in the setting of a mood disturbance. These are characteristics of major depressive disorder with psychotic features.

E. Bipolar I disorder [incorrect]. This diagnosis requires a history of at least one episode of mania.

6-A

A. Malingering [correct]. The patient's primary motivation for self-harm seems to have been the secondary gain of getting out of jail. The deliberate feigning or production of illness or injury prompted by secondary gain is most congruent with a diagnosis of malingering.

B. Factitious disorder [incorrect]. This diagnosis features the deliberate production of feigning of injury or illness with the chief motivation of assuming the sick role, not for any secondary gain.

C. Borderline personality disorder [incorrect]. This condition is frequently associated with self-harming behaviors, but these typically occur in the context of emotional dysregulation and perceived abandonment.

D. Sexual masochism [incorrect]. This involves sexual arousal associated with being humiliated or made to suffer by another person.

E. Trichotillomania [incorrect]. This specifically focuses on repetitive plucking or pulling of hair. No other form of self-harm or injury is involved.

7-D

A. Fluoxetine [incorrect]. This does not have MAO inhibitor activity.

B. Bupropion [incorrect]. This does not have MAO inhibitor activity.

C. Buspirone [incorrect]. This does not have MAO inhibitor activity.

D. Tranylcypromine [correct]. The patient is suffering from a hypertensive crisis, most likely caused by an interaction between an MAO inhibitor and a substance high in tyramine (eg, Chianti wine, aged cheese). Of the agents listed, only tranylcypromine has MAO inhibitor activity.

E. Nortriptyline [incorrect]. This does not have MAO inhibitor activity.

8-C

A. Sodium and bicarbonate [incorrect]. Although electrolytes such as sodium and bicarbonate can be affected in states of malnutrition, hypomagnesemia and hypophosphatemia are the hallmarks of refeeding syndrome.

B. Potassium and chloride [incorrect]. Although electrolytes such as potassium and chloride can be affected in states of malnutrition, hypomagnesemia and hypophosphatemia are the hallmarks of refeeding syndrome.

C. Magnesium and phosphate [correct]. The patient is suffering from refeeding syndrome due to too-rapid introduction of calories in the setting of anorexia nervosa. Refeeding syndrome is caused by the sudden cellular reuptake of magnesium and phosphate, leading to dangerously low serum levels of these electrolytes. Refeeding syndrome can present with a variety of cardiac and neurological symptoms, and it can be fatal. Although other electrolytes can be affected in states of malnutrition, hypomagnesemia and hypophosphatemia are the hallmarks of refeeding syndrome.

D. Calcium and chloride [incorrect]. Although electrolytes such as calcium and chloride can be affected in states of malnutrition, hypomagnesemia and hypophosphatemia are the hallmarks of refeeding syndrome.

E. BUN and creatinine [incorrect]. Although electrolytes such as BUN and creatinine can be affected in states of malnutrition, hypomagnesemia and hypophosphatemia are the hallmarks of refeeding syndrome.

9-A

A. Honor the patient's wishes and allow him to go home [correct]. Despite the diagnosis of mild Alzheimer disease, the patient is consistent in his choice, displays an understanding of his situation, is able to foresee the downstream consequences of the decision he is making, and expresses a rationale for it. As such, he has the capacity to make choices regarding his treatment.

B. Defer the decision to the daughter due to the diagnosis of Alzheimer dementia [incorrect]. Although the daughter's concerns are understandable, a health care proxy is enacted only in cases where the patient is found to lack capacity to make a decision for himself or herself.

C. Proceeding with surgery on the basis of the ethical principle of beneficence [incorrect]. Proceeding with the surgery against the wishes of a patient with the capacity to refuse would be grounds for professional and legal action.

D. Keep the patient in the hospital for another week to see if he changes his mind [incorrect]. Holding this patient in the hospital against his wishes would be grounds for professional and legal action.

E. Ask the hospital attorney to file for a court-appointed guardian for the patient [incorrect]. Court-appointed guardians are sought in cases where the patient does not have capacity to make his or her own decision and there is no reasonable source of a substituted decision (eg, close family member).

10-B

A. Document the error in the chart [incorrect]. Although this is an important step, it does not supersede the responsibility to inform the patient.

B. Inform the patient of the error [correct]. When confidentiality is breached, the physician's chief duty is to inform the patient of the breach. Although documenting the error in the chart, attempting to ascertain the destination of the misplaced information, and instituting safeguards against future mistakes are important, they do not supersede the responsibility to inform the patient.

C. Ascertain the destination of the erroneous fax [incorrect]. Contacting the recipient of the erroneous fax is an important step to determine the destination of the misplaced information but does not supersede the responsibility to inform the patient.

D. Institute a more reliable system of transmitting medical information [incorrect]. Although instituting safeguards against future mistakes are important, this step does not supersede the responsibility to inform the patient.

E. Request another signed release from the patient [incorrect]. There is no indication for an additional signed release.

11-E

A. Fluoxetine [incorrect]. This agent is an antidepressant and is likely to exacerbate mania.

B. Phenelzine [incorrect]. This agent is an antidepressant and is likely to exacerbate mania.

C. Nortriptyline [incorrect]. This agent is an antidepressant and is likely to exacerbate mania.

D. Bupropion [incorrect]. This agent is an antidepressant and is likely to exacerbate mania.

E. Lithium [correct]. The patient is presenting with symptoms of mania, which requires treatment with a mood-stabilizer such as lithium.

12-C

A. GAD [incorrect]. This condition features excessive anxiety or worry about a wide range of issues and is not associated with a specific stimulus.

B. Avoidant personality disorder [incorrect]. This condition consists of a broad pervasive pattern of social avoidance, including intimate relationships.

C. Social phobia [correct]. This disorder is marked by a persistent fear of embarrassment or scrutiny in group settings, producing symptoms of anxiety that the patient typically realizes are out of proportion to the stimulus.

D. Panic disorder with agoraphobia [incorrect]. This condition requires the presence of panic attacks (periods of intense fear associated with multiple symptoms of autonomic arousal, typically peaking in 10 minutes). Agoraphobia is fear of having a panic attack in a place or situation from which escape might be difficult or where assistance might be unavailable.

E. Specific phobia [incorrect]. This condition is characterized by fear of a specific object or situation, and the fear is similarly recognized as unreasonable. Fear of embarrassment or scrutiny in social situations is, however, considered a diagnostically separate entity.

13-D

A. Call the police to arrest the husband [incorrect]. Doing this without the explicit permission of the patient would be a violation of her confidentiality. Informing the authorities without permission can be acceptable in cases of child abuse or elder abuse.

B. Refer the patient and her husband to couple's therapy [incorrect]. Active domestic abuse is widely considered a contraindication to couple's therapy.

C. Tell the patient that spousal abuse is grounds for divorce and she should leave her husband [incorrect]. Care should be taken to maintain a supportive and nonconfrontational tone with the patient, because leaving the abuser may entail a broad variety of consequences, including increased violence, homelessness, and loss of social supports.

D. Educate the patient about domestic violence and the options available to maintain her safety [correct]. It is important to appreciate the sense of fear and risk of reprisal faced by the patient as she considers leaving an abusive relationship. Information should be provided in a reassuring, nonjudgmental fashion, with an emphasis on safety and confidentiality.

E. Provide psychiatric hospitalization to the patient for her own protection [incorrect]. With no evidence of psychiatric illness, involuntary psychiatric hospitalization should not be considered.

14-A

A. Fetishism [correct]. This is characterized by the use of nonliving objects for sexual arousal. Women's clothing, undergarments, and shoes are common examples.

B. Transvestic fetishism [incorrect]. This involves cross-dressing in women's clothes for sexual arousal.

C. Frotteurism [incorrect]. This features rubbing against an unsuspecting individual for sexual arousal.

D. Exhibitionism [incorrect]. This is characterized by sexual arousal derived from the exposure of genitalia to an unsuspecting stranger.

E. Paraphilia not otherwise specified [incorrect]. This is reserved for paraphilias that are not better described by one of the other diagnostic categories.

15-B

A. Olanzapine [incorrect]. This agent is not commonly associated with agranulocytosis.

B. Clozapine [correct]. Agranulocytosis is a dangerous adverse effect of treatment with clozapine that requires frequent monitoring of WBC.

C. Quetiapine [incorrect]. This agent is not commonly associated with agranulocytosis.

D. Aripiprazole [incorrect]. This agent is not commonly associated with agranulocytosis.

E. Risperidone [incorrect]. This agent is not commonly associated with agranulocytosis.

16-E

    A. Benztropine [incorrect]. This agent, available as Cogentin, is an anticholinergic medication that can be used both for the prevention and treatment of dystonic reactions. Anticholinergic agents have little efficacy in the treatment of akathisia.

    B. Diphenhydramine [incorrect]. This agent, available as Benadryl, is an example of an anticholinergic agent. Anticholinergic agents have little efficacy in the treatment of akathisia.

    C. Increased risperidone [incorrect]. Because risperidone is likely the agent causing the akathisia, increasing the dosage is likely to exacerbate it further.

    D. Haloperidol [incorrect]. This agent is a neuroleptic. Although a change in the patient's medication regimen may eventually be indicated, neuroleptics are not used for the acute treatment of akathisia.

    E. Propranolol [correct]. The patient is presenting with symptoms of akathisia, likely in response to the neuroleptic risperidone. The first-line treatment for akathisia is the use of a beta-blocker such as propranolol.

17-A

    A. Potassium and magnesium [correct]. Hypokalemia and hypomagnesemia (along with older age, female gender, bradycardia, LVH, and cardiac ischemia) are risk factors for prolonged QTc and torsades de pointes. Only potassium and magnesium are specifically linked to QTc prolongation.

    B. Sodium and calcium [incorrect]. These substances are not specifically linked to QTc prolongation.

    C. Phosphate and bicarbonate [incorrect]. These substances are not specifically linked to QTc prolongation.

    D. BUN and creatinine [incorrect]. These substances are not specifically linked to QTc prolongation.

    E. Glucose and chloride [incorrect]. These substances are not specifically linked to QTc prolongation.

18-C

    A. GABA [incorrect]. PCP does not act primarily via the GABAergic receptor.

    B. Acetylcholine [incorrect]. PCP does not act primarily via the acetylcholine receptor.

    C. NMDA [correct]. PCP acts primarily via antagonism at the PCP receptor of the ion channel-gated NMDA receptor complex.

D. Norepinephrine [incorrect]. PCP does not act primarily via the norepinephrine receptor.

E. Serotonin [incorrect]. PCP does not act primarily via the serotonin receptor.

19-E

A. ADHD [incorrect]. This disorder is characterized primarily by symptoms of inattention and hyperactivity. Although this can frequently lead to disruptive behavior in the school environment, ADHD does not incorporate the deliberate violation of the rights of others seen in conduct disorder.

B. Oppositional defiant disorder [incorrect]. This condition is distinguished by predominantly defiant and hostile behaviors without serious violations of social norms or the rights of others.

C. Antisocial personality disorder [incorrect]. Like oppositional defiant disorder, this condition involves an inflexible, maladaptive, and pervasive pattern of disregard for the rights of others. However, no personality disorder can be diagnosed in an individual younger than 18 years of age.

D. Narcissistic personality disorder [incorrect]. This condition comprises a pervasive pattern of grandiosity, need for admiration, and lack of empathy. No personality disorder can be diagnosed in an individual younger than 18 years of age.

E. Conduct disorder [correct]. As seen with this patient, conduct disorder is marked by a consistent pattern of violation of the rights of others, or of major societal rules, including behaviors of aggression, destruction of property, deceit, and theft.

20-E

A. Disulfiram [incorrect]. This agent, known as Antabuse, may be useful in maintaining long-term abstinence from alcohol, but it does not treat the acute withdrawal syndrome.

B. Citalopram [incorrect]. This agent, available as Celexa, or other antidepressants can be used to treat depression or anxiety disorders that are frequently comorbid with alcohol dependence, but it does not address the acute withdrawal syndrome.

C. Naltrexone [incorrect]. This agent, available as ReVia, may be useful in maintaining long-term abstinence from alcohol, but it does not treat the acute withdrawal syndrome.

D. Acamprosate [incorrect]. This agent, available as Campral, may be useful in maintaining long-term abstinence from alcohol, but it does not treat the acute withdrawal syndrome.

E. Chlordiazepoxide [correct]. The patient is suffering the symptoms of alcohol withdrawal, and administration of a cross-tolerant substance (a benzodiazepine or barbiturate) is required to forestall possible progression to seizure and death. Of the agents listed, chlordiazepoxide (Librium) is the only example of a benzodiazepine. None of the substances listed is a barbiturate.

credits

Becker KL, Bilezikian JP, Brenner WJ, et al. *Principles and Practice of Endocrinology and Metabolism.* 3rd ed. Philadelphia, PA: Lippincott Williams & Wilkins, 2001. Fig. 120-1 (24-1).

Berek JS. *Berek & Novak's Gynecology.* 14th ed. Philadelphia, PA: Lippincott Williams & Wilkins, 2005. Fig. 26.14 (41-1).

Eisenberg RL. *Clinical Imaging: An Atlas of Differential Diagnosis.* 4th ed. Philadelphia, PA: Lippincott Williams & Wilkins, 2002. Fig. B 20-1 (19-1).

Greer JP, Foerster J, et al. *Wintrobe's Clinical Hematology.* 11th ed. Philadelphia, PA: Lippincott Williams & Wilkins, 2003. Fig. 29.9 (14-1).

Humes HD, et al. *Kelley's Textbook of Internal Medicine.* 4th ed. Philadelphia, PA: Lippincott Williams & Wilkins, 2001. Fig. 82.6 (40-1).

McMillan JA, Fergin RD, et al. *Oski's Pediatrics: Principles and Practice.* 4th ed. Philadelphia, PA: Lippincott Williams & Wilkins, 2006. Fig. 55.5 (49-1).

Mulholland MW, Lillemoe KD, Doherty GM, et al. *Greenfield's Surgery: Scientific Principles & Practice.* 4th ed. Philadelphia, PA: Lippincott Williams & Wilkins, 2005. Fig. 73.31 (23-1).

Rowland LP. *Merritt's Neurology.* 11th ed. Philadelphia, PA: Lippincott Williams & Wilkins, 2005. Fig. 113.3 (39-1).

Sadock BJ, Sadock VA. *Kaplan & Sadock's Synopsis of Psychiatry.* 9th ed. Philadelphia, PA: Lippincott Williams & Wilkins, 2004. Fig. 36.4.18-1 (32-1).

case list

NEUROLOGY

1. Delirium
2. Dementia
3. Wernicke-Korsakoff Syndrome
4. Lewy Body Dementia (LBD)
5. Tourette Disorder
6. Complex Partial Seizures (CPS)

ADJUSTMENT DISORDER

7. Adjustment Disorder

ANXIETY DISORDER

8. Specific Phobia
9. Generalized Anxiety Disorder (GAD)
10. Obsessive-Compulsive Disorder (OCD)
11. Panic Disorder
12. Post-Traumatic Stress Disorder (PTSD)
13. Social Phobia

CHILD PSYCHIATRY

14. Attention-Deficit Hyperactivity Disorder (ADHD)
15. Autism
16. Child Sexual Abuse
17. Conduct Disorder
18. Sleep Terror Disorder
19. Pica
20. Asperger Disorder
21. Separation Anxiety Disorder
22. Oppositional Defiant Disorder (ODD)

PSYCHOPHARMACOLOGY

23. Alcohol Dependence
24. Cannabis Intoxication
25. Cocaine Abuse
26. Alcohol Withdrawal
27. Lysergic Acid Diethylamide Intoxication
28. Opiate Withdrawal
29. Phencyclidine Intoxication
30. Opiate Intoxication
31. Amphetamine Intoxication
32. Lithium Toxicity
33. Hypertensive Crisis
34. Tardive Dyskinesia (TD)
35. Agranulocytosis
36. Neuroleptic Malignant Syndrome (NMS)
37. Serotonin Syndrome
38. Akathisia
39. Acute Dystonia
40. QTc Prolongation

EATING DISORDERS

41. Anorexia Nervosa
42. Bulimia Nervosa

ETHICS

43. Capacity
44. Disclosure of Teen Pregnancy
45. Fetal Neglect
46. Withdrawal of Care
47. Patient–Doctor Confidentiality
48. Tarasoff Decision
49. Withholding Treatment

FACTIOUS DISORDERS

50. Factitious Disorder

51. Malingering

GENDER DISORDERS

52. Gender Identity Disorder

MOOD DISORDERS

53. Bereavement

54. Bipolar I Disorder

55. Mood Disorder Due to a General Medical Condition

56. Major Depressive Disorder

57. Dysthymic Disorder

58. Bipolar II Disorder

59. Seasonal Affective Disorder (SAD)

60. Postpartum Depression

PERSONALITY DISORDERS

61. Antisocial Personality Disorder

62. Borderline Personality Disorder

63. Schizoid Personality Disorder

64. Schizotypal Personality Disorder

65. Narcissistic Personality Disorder

66. Histrionic Personality Disorder

PSYCHOTIC DISORDERS

67. Brief Psychotic Disorder

68. Delusional Disorder

69. Schizophrenia

70. Schizoaffective Disorder

SOMATOFORM DISORDERS

71. Body Dysmorphic Disorder (BDD)

72. Conversion Disorder

73. Hypochondriasis

74. Somatization Disorder

PARAPHILIAS

75. Kleptomania

76. Trichotillomania

77. Transvestic Fetishism

78. Frotteurism

ABUSE

79. Domestic Violence

80. Elder Abuse

index